Cases in Neurogenic
Communicative Disorders
A Workbook

Second Edition

Cases in Neurogenic Communicative Disorders

A Workbook

Second Edition

by

James P. Dworkin, Ph.D.
Professor, Department of Otolaryngology
Wayne State University
School of Medicine
Detroit, Michigan

and

David E. Hartman, Ph.D.
Head, Speech Pathology, Department of Neurology
Gundersen Clinic, Ltd., and Gundersen Medical Foundation
La Crosse, Wisconsin

SINGULAR PUBLISHING GROUP, INC.
San Diego, California

Singular Publishing Group, Inc.
4284 41st Street
San Diego, California 92105-1197

® 1994 by Singular Publishing Group, Inc.

Typeset in 9½/11½ Chelmsford Medium by House Graphics
Printed in the United States of America by BookCrafters

Library of Congress Cataloging-in-Publication Data
Dworkin, James Paul.
    Cases in neurogenic communicative disorders: a workbook / by
James P. Dworkin and David E. Hartman.—2nd ed.
        p.   cm.
    Includes bibliographical references and index.
    ISBN 1-56593-264-1
    1. Language disorders—Case studies. 2. Speech disorders—Case
studies.   I. Hartman, David E.   II. Title.
RC423.D86   1993
616.85'509—dc20   93-30762
                                                            CIP

Contents

Preface

In the second edition of our book, we have attempted to introduce the readership to additional cases, based on our professional experiences, and an updated bibliography. We felt that a revision of the text was necessary in view of the advances and changes in health care that confront us and with which we deal daily. The format of the book remains unchanged; we have added new information where relevant and have retained that which remains current.

Medical speech-language pathology is now recognized as a specialty area of practice whose clinicians focus primarily on neurologic and laryngologic disorders of communication. In recognition of this area of practice, several special interest groups sponsored by the American Speech-Language Hearing Association have been formed. The Academy of Neurologic Communication Disorders and Sciences and the journals of *Voice* and *Medical Speech-Language Pathology* also reflect this continued growth and interest.

Health care reform will offer new challenges to those of us who practice within the medical community. Cost containment and accountability are perhaps the most pressing issues influencing what we do and why, when, and how we do it. New directions for differential diagnosis and treatment have begun to orchestrate our attention to these demands; we hope this text will assist medical speech-language pathologists and physicians in this process.

We again express our gratitude and appreciation to our mentors and colleagues from whom we have learned how to separate the wheat from the chaff and where to go from there. We are especially indebted to our loving families—you needed to be there. Finally, as always, we thank our patients, from whom we learn and grow in order to help them further.

JPD

DEH

Instructions

This textbook is divided into two sections. The first section introduces a brief overview of the speech-language and neurologic characteristics of the various types of neurogenic communicative disorders. The description of the disorders and their neurologic substrates should not be considered all-inclusive, but rather should be viewed as a guide for the analyses of the cases presented in Section 2. Review of the first section should precede examination of the individual Case Studies.

The second section presents randomized case histories. A brief clinical history and description of the neurologic and speech-language signs and symptoms are provided at the beginning of each case. The task for the reader, once the history of a case is read, is to determine the speech-language diagnosis of the case, as well as to make inferences regarding the medical diagnosis and the site of lesion, prior to turning the page for the answer. A worksheet (like that on page xii) and blank illustrations (see the examples on pages xiii-xvi) are provided for each case, to enable the reader to record the symptoms and signs that appear diagnostically salient and to sketch the suspected site of lesion. A discussion and illustrated site of lesion follows. For illustrative purposes, the authors have exercised a degree of artistic license for identifying lesion sites on the schematic drawings of the brain.

A bibliography and an index listing each Case Study by type of communicative disorder and page number for each reference appear at the end of the text. Since many of the cases presented benefited from speech-language intervention, the reader is referred to Johns's (1985) text, *Clinical Management of Neurogenic Communicative Disorders*, Second Edition and Dworkin's (1991) book *Motor Speech Disorders: A Treatment Guide* for specific treatment strategies that may be relevant for comparable cases. For those readers who are interested in audio samples, a screening test format for focal neurogenic disorders of communication, and what to look and listen for in patients who have aphasia, apraxia of speech, and dysarthria, an article by Hartman and Dworkin (1993) may prove useful.

The cases in this text are based on the medical records of actual patients. It is important to keep in mind, as these cases are reviewed, that in clinical practice an unequivocal diagnosis may not always be reached for each patient. Certain neurologic conditions are marked by changing speech and language characteristics that must be monitored over time before logical conclusions can be drawn. Most of the cases presented here, however, were selected because they lent themselves to definitive diagnosis.

Worksheet

Salient symptoms/signs	Test results	Impressions

This worksheet is to be used for recording relevant diagnostic observations. The blank illustration is to be used for identifying and sketching the suspected site of lesion(s). These steps should be completed prior to turning to the Impressions and illustrated site of lesion.

The left cerebral hemisphere and macroscopic representation of the major cortical centers for speech and language.

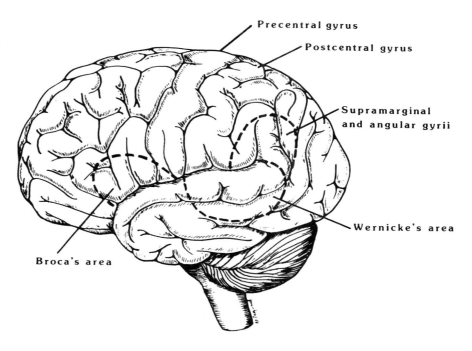

Precentral gyrus

Postcentral gyrus

Supramarginal and angular gyrii

Wernicke's area

Broca's area

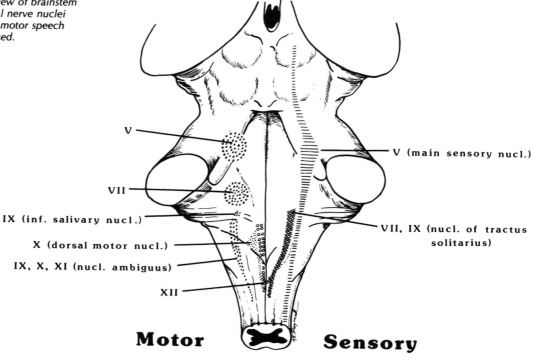

*Posterior view of brainstem
with cranial nerve nuclei
subserving motor speech
superimposed.*

V

V (main sensory nucl.)

VII

IX (inf. salivary nucl.)

X (dorsal motor nucl.)

IX, X, XI (nucl. ambiguus)

XII

VII, IX (nucl. of tractus
solitarius)

Motor   **Sensory**

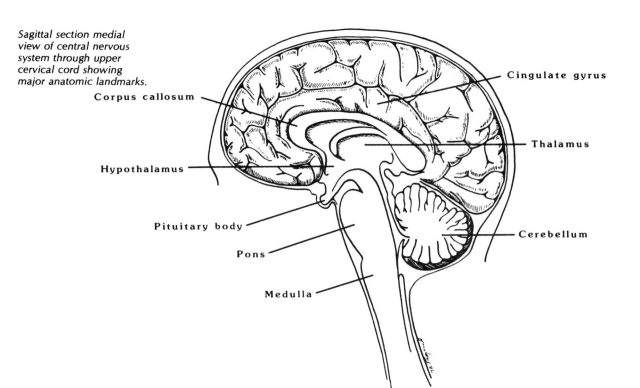

Sagittal section medial view of central nervous system through upper cervical cord showing major anatomic landmarks.

Corpus callosum

Cingulate gyrus

Thalamus

Hypothalamus

Pituitary body

Pons

Cerebellum

Medulla

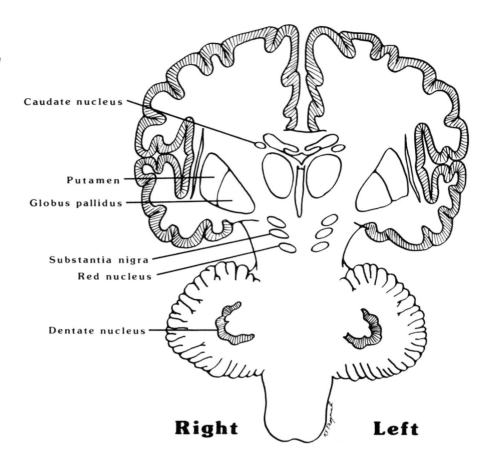

Coronal section medial view of central nervous system through brainstem showing important subcortical centers for motor speech control.

Caudate nucleus

Putamen

Globus pallidus

Substantia nigra

Red nucleus

Dentate nucleus

Right

Left

Cases in Neurogenic Communicative Disorders
A Workbook

1 Review of Neurogenic Communicative Disorders

Language and Speech: Definitions

For the purposes of this text, language and speech will be defined as follows:

Language involves comprehension, formulation, and utilization of words and symbols, depending upon the integrity of the central language processor, an area of the dominant (usually the left) cerebral hemisphere corresponding roughly to the midposterior temporal, parietal (including the angular and supramarginal gyri), and anterior occipital lobe areas.

Speech, as a motor act, involves the production of sounds and meaningful sequences of sounds for the transmission of language. Speech production is dependent upon: (1) the motor speech programmer, an area of the dominant (usually the left) cerebral hemisphere corresponding roughly to Brodmann's area 44 on the inferior-lateral-posterior frontal lobe (Broca's area) and supplemental motor cortex; and (2) the speech effectors, consisting of the motor strips bilaterally; extrapyramidal and pyramidal tracts; subcortical nuclei, including the basal ganglia; the brainstem and cerebellum; and the cranial and spinal nerves that directly subserve motor speech control. The structural integrity of the speech mechanism is understood to be normal in this definition.

Etiology of Neurogenic Communicative Disorders

Damage to the central nervous system, peripheral nervous system or both may cause different types and degrees of speech-language disturbances, the characteristics of which usually depend upon the areas affected and the underlying neuropathologic cause. For example, trauma may result in speech-language and behavioral signs that are consistent with diffuse impairment of the nervous system. A disturbance or alteration in blood flow caused by cerebrovascular accident can produce specific speech-language impairment consistent with the site of involvement. Neoplasms may produce variable speech-language signs as they replace or displace neural and vascular tissue.

Other causative agents may include: (1) infectious processes such as meningitis; (2) toxicity, as in chronic alcoholism; (3) interrupted oxygen to the nervous system; (4) metabolic deficiencies such as low serum sodium; (5) degenerative and demyelinating diseases including amyotrophic lateral sclerosis, Huntington's disease, multiple sclerosis; (6) trauma; and (7) disorders for which no cause can be determined (idiopathic). To remember these causes, the acronym **VITAMIN D** may be useful, with each letter representing a possible cause: **V** (vascular), **I** (infectious, ictal), **T** (traumatic or toxic), **A** (anoxic), **M** (metabolic), **I** (idiopathic, iatrogenic), **N** (neoplastic), **D** (degenerative, demyelinating, or developmental).

There are various ways of classifying neurogenic disorders of communication. We have chosen the model proposed by Mayo Clinic, which recognizes five primary disorders: aphasia, generalized intellectual impairment or dementia, language of confusion, apraxia of speech, and the dysarthrias. To a certain degree each of the disorders has localizing value within the central or peripheral nervous systems.

The text views each of the disorders from a perceptual basis-that which is seen and heard. The reader should recognize, however, that physiological and acoustic measures are frequently tantamount to accurate diagnosis and effective treatment. The disorders are summarized in Table 1.

Table 1. *Type of Neurogenic Communicative Disorders: Cardinal Signs and Lesion Sites*

Disorder	Site of lesion	Articulation	Phonation	Resonation	Respiration	Prosody	Language	Language/ Intellect
Dysarthria	CNS/PNS	X	X	X	X	X		
Apraxia of speech	Unilateral-cerebral	X				X		
Aphasia	Unilateral-cerebral						X	
Generalized intellectual impairment/ dementia	Bilateral-cerebral							X
*Confused language	Unilateral R-cerebral, or bilateral-cerebral							X

*Can evolve into generalized intellectual impairment if present on a chronic basis.

Aphasia *Aphasia* is characterized by impaired comprehension, formulation, and functional use of language. The disorder crosses all language modalities including listening (auditory comprehension and retention), reading, writing, and speaking. The patient with aphasia may have difficulty understanding individual words, phrases, and sentences. Difficulty in recalling an appropriate word, such as the name of a person, place, or thing, may result in the substitution of an associated or erroneous word or term. Auditory retention difficulties, such as impairment in processing a sequence of linguistic elements, may result in nonmeaningful verbal or written responses. The organization of sentences, both spoken and written, may be syntactically incorrect and marked by word omissions and word and phrase repetitions. Written words may be misspelled; linguistic items may be used beyond their point of usefulness (perseveration); verbalization may be nonsensical (jargon); and new words may be created (neologisms).

Aphasia itself is not the result of, nor is it chiefly characterized by, sensory and motor deficiencies such as hearing loss, blindness, paralysis, hypertonia, or incoordination. Sensory-motor disturbances, however, frequently do coexist with aphasia.

Aphasia usually results from a lesion in one or more areas of the dominant (left in most cases) cerebral hemisphere. These may include: (1) Wernicke's area in the superoposterior zone of the temporal lobe; (2) arcuate fasciculi that interconnect Broca's and Wernicke's areas; and (3) Parietal-occipital lobe areas, including the angular and supramarginal gyri. A lesion in Broca's area may not produce true aphasia, as defined above, but, rather, difficulty planning and initiating the speech act.

Aphasia must be differentiated from generalized intellectual impairment (dementia), language of confusion, and apraxia of speech.

Generalized Intellectual Impairment *Generalized intellectual impairment,* also known as *dementia,* is characterized by gross, progressive deterioration in all cognitive skills including language. The language deficit, which crosses all modalities, is generally proportionate to the deterioration of other mental functions—a finding that is not true for specific language disorders such as aphasia. Impaired memory affects attention and retention as cognitive tasks become more complex. Greater attention is required to obtain meaning from complex stimuli. Abstract thought and reasoning are affected. The patient may speak less often, frequently offering concrete, perseverative verbalizations.

Although focal neurogenic communicative disorders, including aphasia, may occur with generalized intellectual impairment, the primary sign is reduced verbal and nonverbal intellectual functioning. To help substantiate the intellectual component, a neuropsychological evaluation is frequently necessary.

Generalized intellectual impairment is usually described as being diffuse or multifocal due to brain pathology involving both cerebral hemispheres.

Language of Confusion The noteworthy and distinguishing signs of *confused language* include confabulation (utterances rendered without respect to truth); disorientation to time, place, and person; faulty memory and conceptualization; and impaired understanding and recognition of the environment. Verbalizations in response to simple and specific stimuli are generally grammatically and semantically intact. However, more complex and less specific stimuli can render confabulatory responses, even though sentence structure remains relatively intact.

Intellectual functioning may be difficult to determine for the confused patient due to the confabulatory nature and irrelevance of responses to verbal and nonverbal stimuli. Other neurogenic communicative disorders may coexist with confused language, but are not components of the basic disorder.

Diffuse or multifocal bilateral cerebral pathology, usually traumatically induced, is considered the primary cause of confused language. However, with unilateral focal involvement, typically of the right hemisphere, confusion may also be observed.

Apraxia of Speech *Apraxia of speech* is predominantly characterized by faulty programming of speech musculature for the sequential movements necessary for ongoing speech production. The patient with apraxia of speech gropes for accurate articulatory postures, trying to place the tongue, jaws, lips and soft palate, and occasionally the vocal folds in the correct position for the production of a given sound or sequence of sounds.

The majority of articulation errors are unpredictable and inconsistent. They include: (1) substitutions, whereby one sound is substituted for another; (2) additions, in which an extra sound is added to a word; (3) omissions, in which a sound is left out of a word; (4) transpositions, whereby sounds or syllables are inverted; (5) repetitions, whereby sounds or words are repeated; and (6) prolongations, in which a sound is sustained beyond a reasonable limit.

As the articulatory task becomes longer and more complex, the patient with apraxia of speech may exhibit more production errors. With repeated trials, however, a particular error may improve. The rhythm or prosody of speech is frequently disturbed and therefore has a halting, stuttering quality. Frequently the patient is aware of speech production errors but can do little to correct them. Automatic speech (common utterances, obscenity, etc.) is generally better than volitional (purposeful) speech.

Patients with apraxia of speech frequently demonstrate an associated oral apraxia, and as such have difficulty performing volitional non-speech tasks with the tongue, lips, and cheeks. It is important to note that these apraxic disturbances are not the result of significant weakness, slowness, incoordination, or altered tone of the speech musculature; rather, their origin is at a higher programming level of speech production.

Language deficits are not inherent components of apraxia of speech. However, apraxia of speech frequently occurs with aphasia, thereby rendering a language disturbance as well.

The site of lesion resulting in apraxia of speech is usually ascribed to Broca's convolution in the inferolateral-posterior frontal lobe of the dominant cerebral hemisphere, or dominant supplemental motor cortex.

Dysarthria

Dysarthria represents a group of speech disorders characterized by disturbances in speech muscular control due to paralysis, paresis, weakness, slowness, incoordination, and/or altered tone. One or more of the motor processes of speech production, including respiration, phonation, articulation, resonance, and prosody (speech rhythm), may be involved. In severe dysarthria, a patient's speech may be rendered virtually unintelligible, as the speech musculature cannot be activated with normal speed, precision, coordination, or timing.

In mild dysarthria, the only sign of neuromuscular involvement may be chronic hoarseness, imprecise articulation, hypernasality, or respiratory difficulties. Contrary to the unpredictability and inconsistency of articulation errors noted in apraxia of speech, dysarthric speech errors tend to be regular and consistent. Language impairment is not a component of dysarthria; dysarthria needs to be differentiated from apraxia of speech.

Seven major types of dysarthria have been identified: (1) flaccid, (2) spastic, (3) unilateral upper motor neuron (UUMN), (4) ataxic, (5) hypokinetic, (6) hyperkinetic, and (7) mixed. Each can be described in terms of site of lesion and speech symptomology.

Flaccid Dysarthria

Unilateral or bilateral damage to cranial or spinal nerves (lower motor neurons, LMN) that innervate the respiratory, phonatory, articulatory, and resonatory musculature results in flaccid dysarthria. Direct damage to speech musculature may also cause this motor speech disorder.

Neuromuscular signs include paralysis or paresis, hypotonicity, atrophy, fasciculations, and hypoactive reflexes of involved musculature. To varying degrees, all types of movements—volitional, automatic, and reflexive—are involved. These symptoms are diagnosed medically as *bulbar palsy.*

Speech characteristics depend on which LMN's are damaged, and the site and extent of involvement. In the case of involvement of a single nerve (mononeuropathy), the lesion usually occurs somewhere along the course of the nerve. Involvement of more than one nerve (polyneuropathy) may be due to lesions in the brainstem or spinal cord, where nuclei originate and are in close proximity. Generally, a polyneuropathy is characterized by more widespread neuromuscular impairment than is a mononeuropathy.

Hypernasality and nasal emission may result from lesions of the IX and X cranial nerves, which supply the velopharyngeal musculature. Imprecise and slow-labored articulatory movements may be due to damage to the VII, XII, and V cranial nerves, which, respectively, supply the facial, lingual, and mandibular musculature. Hoarse, gurgly, breathy phonation may occur when the recurrent and superior laryngeal branches of the Xth cranial nerve, which supply the laryngeal musculature, are involved. Poor respiratory support for speech may occur because of damage to those spinal nerves that supply the muscles of respiration, or to the Xth cranial nerve. The XIth cranial nerve must be intact to keep the head, and therefore the vocal tract, upright.

Spastic Dysarthria

Bilateral damage to those upper motor neurons (UMN) that synapse with cranial nerve nuclei that supply the speech musculature, viz, corticobulbar tract fibers, results in varying degrees of *spastic dysarthria*.

Neuromuscular signs include paresis, weakness, hypertonicity, and hyperactive reflexes below the level of the lesion. In some individuals, emotional incontinence characterized by unprovoked, short outbursts of crying or laughing is noted. These symptoms are diagnosed medically as *pseudobulbar palsy*.

Speech characteristics include imprecise articulation; variable hypernasality, with "wail-like" slowed speaking rate and nasal air emission; strain-strangled phonation; and reduced respiratory support for speech. Unilateral corticobulbar tract damage produces weakness of the contralateral musculature, particularly of the face and tongue, with resultant articulation impairment. The speech appears almost flaccid or ataxic like.

UUMN Dysarthria

Unilateral damage to the corticobulbar tracts anywhere along the tracts' courses from the cortex through the brainstem produces contralateral lower facial and tongue weakness. Speech manifestations include imprecise consonant production, reduced loudness and pitch fluctuation, low pitch, short phrases, and slowed rate. The nature of the phonatory signs—whether compensatory or pathophysiologic—at this time is unclear. Overall speech intelligibility, however, is rarely affected.

Ataxic Dysarthria

Bilateral damage of the cerebellum or its tracts causes incoordination in various parts of the body. When the speech musculature is affected, the result is *ataxic dysarthria*. Unilateral left or bilateral cerebellar damage may impair speech function. Neuromuscular signs of cerebellar involvement include incoordination, wide-based gait, intention tremor, variable hypotonicity, slow and irregular alternate motion of involved musculature, and nystagmus.

Speech characteristics include irregular articulatory imprecision, variably dysrhythmic patterns of contextual speech, harsh vocal quality, and slow and irregular oral alternate and sequential motion rates.

Hypokinetic Dysarthria

Marked degenerative changes in the substantia nigra, in the nuclei of the extrapyramidal system that are functionally related to the basal ganglia, or in the specific extrapyramidal tract fibers that interconnect these nuclei may result in *hypokinetic dysarthria.* This type of dysarthria occurs in individuals with degenerative idiopathic Parkinson's disease, or parkinsonism due to other causes such as certain drugs.

The outstanding neuromuscular signs of Parkinson's disease include cogwheel rigidity, bradykinesia, pill-rolling rest tremor, shuffling gait, flexed truncal posture, and masklike facies.

The major speech characteristics of hypokinetic dysarthria include harsh and breathy phonation; monopitch, monoloudness, and decreased loudness; prolonged syllables; excessive pausing; short rushes of speech; variably fast and slow alternate and sequential motion rates, produced with reduced ranges of movement of involved musculature; alternating fast and slow rates of articulation; and imprecise consonant and vowel production. As the condition progresses, the patient may demonstrate signs of generalized intellectual impairment (dementia).

Hyperkinetic Dysarthria   There are quick, slow, and tremor forms of hyperkinetic dysarthria, which result from lesions of the extrapyramidal system. The quick form includes the speech of chorea while the slow form is observed in individuals with dystonia and some forms of orofacial dyskinesia. Tremor is observed in essential voice tremor. Myoclonus involving the speech musculature may actually be a form of tremor.

Chorea may occur in childhood or adulthood and is primarily a result of damage to the caudate nucleus and putamen (striatum) of the basal ganglia. The childhood form (Sydenham's) is thought to be inflammatory or infectious in origin and is a frequent sequela of rheumatic fever. Patients usually recover from this form of the disease. The adult form (Huntington's disease) is a heredodegenerative and fatal disease that usually appears in adulthood.

Neuromuscular signs of chorea include quick, involuntary, random, and jerky movements of the head, face, limbs, and trunk. Muscle tone varies from states of hypotonia of the extremities to hypertonia of the axial musculature, including the speech mechanism.

Speech characteristics of the dysarthria of chorea include variable rate, inappropriate silences, irregular and imprecise articulation, prolonged phonemes and intervals between words, vocal harshness, monopitch, and monoloudness. Lingual and labial alternate motion rates are variably fast, slow, and interrupted by phonatory arrests. Patients with Huntington's disease frequently experience gross mood swings and intellectual and language deterioration as the disease progresses.

Myoclonic movements involving the peripheral musculature are quick, irregular and unpredictable. However, *palatal-pharyngeal-laryngeal myoclonus* is characterized by relatively predictable and rhythmic contractions between 2-4 Hz of the soft palate, pharynx, larynx, and frequently the base of the tongue. The etiology is thought to be damage to the pathways connecting the red nucleus, olivary bodies of the medulla, and dentate nucleus of the cerebellum. The cardinal sign of palatal-pharyngeal-laryngeal myoclonus is the regular changes (tremor-like) in volume during vowel prolongation that are synchronized with the myoclonic movements. Interestingly, and most important, myoclonic movements of the palate, pharynx, and larynx are present at rest.

Dystonia results from lesions of the striatum and globus pallidus, and is characterized by slow, undulating, twisting, variably prolonged, and involuntary movements of the trunk and proximal parts of the limbs, head, face, tongue, and mandible. Muscle hypertonus is prominent, but tends to wax and wane.

Speech characteristics of the dysarthria of dystonia vary, depending on which structures of the speech mechanism are involved and the degree of their involvement. Characteristics include prolonged intervals between phonemes; variable silences and arrests of phonation; excess loudness variations; breathiness, harshness, monopitch; slow, irregular, and imprecise alternate motion rates of the tongue and lips; and irregular and imprecise consonant and vowel production. Adductor, abductor, or adductor/abductor voice arrest as seen in spasmodic dysphonia may also be a manifestation of focal laryngeal dystonia.

Dyskinesia results from lesions of the basal ganglia, the specific locus of which is not certain. There is considerable controversy regarding the types of dyskinetic movements; however, they are generally described as irregular, and variably quick-jerky to slow-undulating, like those seen in chorea and dystonia, respectively. Movements may be multifocal or focal to the speech mechanism. The use of phenothiazines and similar drugs may cause a gradually developing movement known as *tardive dyskinesia*.

Speech characteristics of the dysarthria of dyskinesia vary between those observed in chorea and dystonia.

Essential voice tremor is a component of the essential (benign, heredofamilial, etc.) tremor syndrome. The site of lesion is unknown, but is thought to be extrapyramidal within the brainstem. Essential voice tremor may occur with or without associated tremor of the hands. It is distinguished from parkinsonian and ataxic tremors by its regularity, relative smoothness, and postural manifestation.

Speech characteristics include rhythmic alterations in loudness ranging from 4-13 Hz, monopitch, and irregular oral alternate and sequential motion rates of any involved musculature. Rhythmic and regular voice arrests on vowel prolongation, accompanied by a choking, strained-harsh, effortful dysphonia, identify the disorder as *spastic (spasmodic) dysphonia* of essential tremor, and distinguish it from the voice signs of focal laryngeal dystonia.

Mixed Dysarthria When multifocal motor system impairment occurs, mixed forms of dysarthria may result. The three most common neurologic diseases in which mixed dysarthria is a component are amyotrophic lateral sclerosis, multiple sclerosis, and Wilson's disease. Mixed dysarthria may also occur in the absence of a specific disease entity, as is often observed in individuals who suffer from diffuse, multifocal nervous system pathology.

A mixed dysarthria reflects the neuromuscular components of the systems involved.

Amyotrophic lateral sclerosis (ALS) is a progressively (degenerative) fatal disease affecting corticobulbar and corticospinal tracts (upper motor neurons) and cranial and spinal nerves (lower motor neurons). Such involvement produces variably spastic-flaccid neuromuscular signs throughout the body.

When the corticobulbar tracts and specific cranial nerve nuclei are involved, a mixed spastic-flaccid (speech) dysarthria results. Comparable signs of spasticity and flaccidity are observed in parts of the body other than the speech musculature when corticospinal tract and spinal nerve nuclei are involved. Since the degeneration of the motor systems is not usually uniform, muscular spasticity or flaccidity may occur alone or in combination, may predominate at any given time, and will range from mild to severe.

Neuromuscular signs include atrophy, fasciculations, weakness, paralysis, spasticity, EMG evidence of denervation, slow and labored alternate motion rates, and hyper/hypoactive reflexes of the affected musculature. In advancing stages of the disease, dysphagia, nasal regurgitation, and respiratory distress usually occur.

Speech characteristics of the dysarthria of ALS include phonation that varies in quality from gurgly (wet)-hoarse to strain-strangled to breathy; monopitch, monoloudness; hypernasality and nasal air emission; imprecise articulation; short phrases; and slow and labored oral alternate and sequential motion rates.

Multiple sclerosis (MS) is an inflammatory condition causing demyelination and scarring of the white matter of the cerebrum, brainstem, cerebellum, and spinal cord. Most individuals afflicted experience exacerbations and remissions of signs and symptoms; the course is generally progressive.

Neuromuscular signs and symptoms are variable and may include wide-based, ataxic gait, generalized hyperreflexia and paresthesias of the extremities, Babinski signs, diplopia, urinary difficulties, and slow and irregular alternate motion rates of affected body parts. Laboratory testing reveals elevated levels of gamma globulin concentrated in the spinal fluid. Occasionally patients present with cortical signs, including speech apraxia, aphasia, and affective disturbances.

Speech characteristics of the spastic-ataxic dysarthria of MS include difficulty with loudness control, vocal harshness, slow and imprecise articulation, impaired emphasis of rate and phrasing, mild hypernasality, and slow and irregular oral alternate and sequential motion rates.

Wilson's disease is a hereditary disorder caused by inadequate copper metabolism and accumulation of copper in the brain, liver, and cornea.

Neuromuscular signs are generally progressive, and include involuntary, nonrhythmic movements of the upper extremities, wide-based gait, reduced range of movement of affected musculature, masklike facies, and slow and irregular alternate motion rates. Laboratory testing reveals low serum-ceruloplasmin and high serum-copper levels.

Speech characteristics of the ataxic-hypokinetic-spastic dysarthria of Wilson's disease include monopitch, monoloudness, vocal harshness, strain-strangled phonation, slow and imprecise articulation, prolonged phonemes, hypernasality, and slow and irregular oral alternate and sequential motion rates. Mixed dysarthrias are also components of progressive supranuclear palsy, multiple systems atrophy, and spino-cerebellar degeneration.

This concludes the review of neurogenic communicative disorders. The following section is comprised of numerous case studies, randomly ordered. The key to solving the diagnosis of each case is the degree to which the reader is familiar with the salient signs and symptoms of various forms of neurologic disease. Information that can be gleaned from the review of a given case should facilitate keener recognition and assessment of other such cases with common backgrounds and clinical histories.

2 Case Studies

27-Year-Old with Speech Difficulty

History   The patient is a 27-year-old male, high school graduate, self-referred for evaluation of communicative function. As he described his complaints concerning articulation, it sounded as though he was a non-native English speaker. His "accent" was unfamiliar. He indicated that since grade school he had struggled with his speech and that he had been frequently ostracized by other children because of his speaking problem. His history was significant in that he had fallen out of a second story window at age seven, but had experienced no ill side affects.

Examination   Language and oral mechanism examinations proved unremarkable. His speech, however, was slow, labored, and imprecise, with significant episodes of intrasyllabic prolongations and pausing within and between words. Numerous anticipatory transpositions of sounds in words and even words within phrases were evident during contextual and contrived speech activities. Overall, articulatory intelligibility was relatively unimpaired. Articulatory-prosodic errors were exacerbated by stuttering-like behaviors, including audible and oral facial groping, false starts and restarts, and improvement with practice (adaptation). Requests to slow and pace his speaking rate resulted in improved intelligibility and articulatory precision. Oral nonspeech movements were normal. Neurologic, neuroimaging (MRI) and neurophysiologic measures (EEG) were normal.

Salient symptoms/signs	Test results	Impressions

This worksheet is to be used for recording relevant diagnostic observations. The blank illustration is to be used for identifying and sketching the suspected site of lesion(s). These steps should be completed prior to turning to the Impressions and illustrated site of lesion.

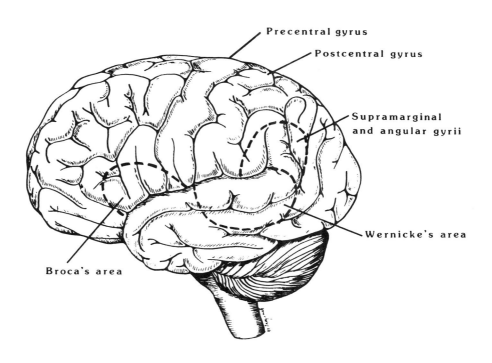

Precentral gyrus

Postcentral gyrus

Supramarginal
and angular gyrii

Wernicke's area

Broca's area

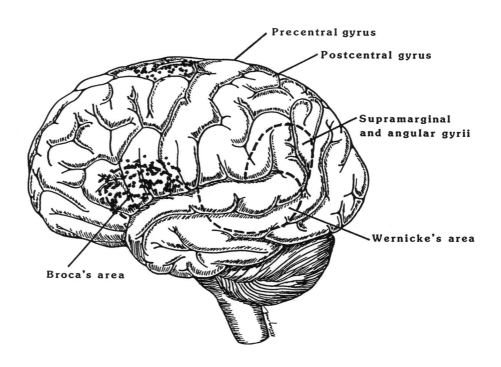

Precentral gyrus

Postcentral gyrus

Supramarginal
and angular gyrii

Wernicke's area

Broca's area

Impressions   Mild dyspraxia of speech, chronic, most likely secondary to closed head injury.

Discussion   The history and clinical signs for this patient support the diagnosis of dyspraxia of speech, although a focal lesion could not be determined by standard neurologic examination. In cases of *chronic* central nervous system damage, particularly when the manifestations are "focal," both neuroimaging and neurophysiologic measures can appear normal. When brain injury occurs in childhood, as in our patient, neuroplasticity and ongoing brain maturation may account for unremarkable neuroimaging findings. Although not available to our patient, a PET (positron emission tomography) scan correlating blood flow with cerebral activity, may have aided in identifying site of lesion. The suspected lesion sites are depicted in the illustration.

This patient's treatment protocol stressed (1) training of slowed, deliberate speaking rate using a metronome to pace articulatory adjustments, (2) evoking and capitalizing on automatic-reactive speech capabilities, (3) using modified melodic intonation therapy techniques to foster sequential articulatory posturing, (4) beginning phonetic training with short, reduplicative utterances, and (5) increasing the length and complexity of utterances as articulation and articulator sequential movement patterns improved. The patient's "accent" may have been the result of vowel distortions, and his stuttering-like behavior (not an uncommon feature in dyspraxia of speech) may have been a co-occurring or compensatory feature of the speech disorder. The vowel distortions were addressed in the phonetic training segment of the treatment plan, with the dysfluency improving with articulation therapy.

65-Year Old Male with Hand Tremors, Hypertonicity, Speech and Swallowing Disturbances

History A 65-year-old male began experiencing a slight, unremitting resting tremor of both hands. Soon after the onset of this symptom he developed mild difficulty with gait, speech, and swallowing, which prompted a complete medical examination. Although a diagnosis was reserved at that time, a drug therapy program was prescribed that included a mixture of trihexyphenidyl (Artane) and carbidopa-levodopa (Sinemet) tablets (25/250 mg.) four times a day. Initially, this program resulted in modest improvement; however, these effects were not sustained, and symptoms gradually worsened over a two-year period. The patient was admitted to the clinic for comprehensive reevaluation.

Examination The patient was alert and cooperative, and used normal language throughout testing.

A slow, shuffling and stooped gait was prominent, but an intermittent tendency to break into a short-stepped trot (festination) was also evident. Attempts to get out of the examination chair unassisted proved unsuccessful. Deep tendon reflexes of the upper limbs were within normal limits, but moderate to severe hypertonicity was observed bilaterally. These signs were accompanied by a phenomenon in which the increased resistance initially felt in each extremity during passive flexing and extending gave way and returned, in an alternating and jerky manner known as *cogwheel rigidity.*

Additionally, a pill-rolling tremor in both hands appeared, in concert with a to-and-fro tremor of the head. Finger tapping and other upper limb alternate motion rate tasks were variably slow-fast, dysrhythmic and imprecise. Lower limb deep reflexes were normal, but severe hypertonicity was detected. Foot tapping and other lower limb alternate motion rate characteristics were analogous to the abnormal upper limb performances.

Bulbar musculature signs and symptoms included: (1) masked facial expression; (2) drooling; (3) hypertonicity of the mandibular, labial, and lingual musculature accompanied by severe limitations in the range, speed, rhythm, and precision of their movements; (4) dysphagia; and (5) dysarthria. The latter condition was chiefly characterized by hoarse-breathy, monopitch, and monoloud phonation; variable slow-fast and imprecise articulation, accompanied by intermittent rushes of syllable and whole-word productions; short phrases; and variable rapid-fire, imprecise, and small-amplitude alternate motion rates of the tongue and lips.

Indirect laryngoscopy suggested incomplete vocal fold adduction. Laboratory studies were normal, except for an elevated serum-uric acid level.

Worksheet

Salient symptoms/signs	Test results	Impressions

This worksheet is to be used for recording relevant diagnostic observations. The blank illustration is to be used for identifying and sketching the suspected site of lesion(s). These steps should be completed prior to turning to the Impressions and illustrated site of lesion.

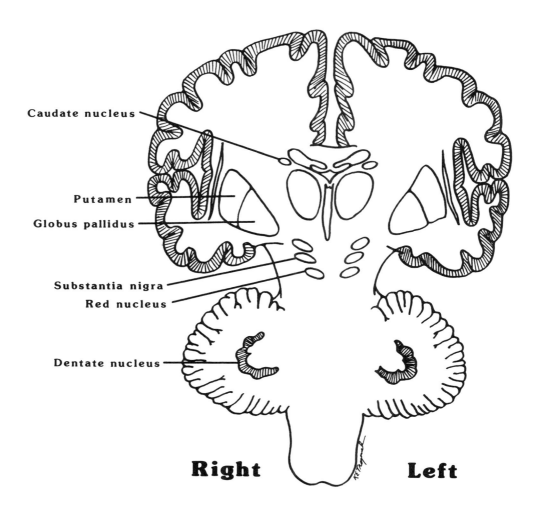

Caudate nucleus

Putamen

Globus pallidus

Substantia nigra

Red nucleus

Dentate nucleus

Right

Left

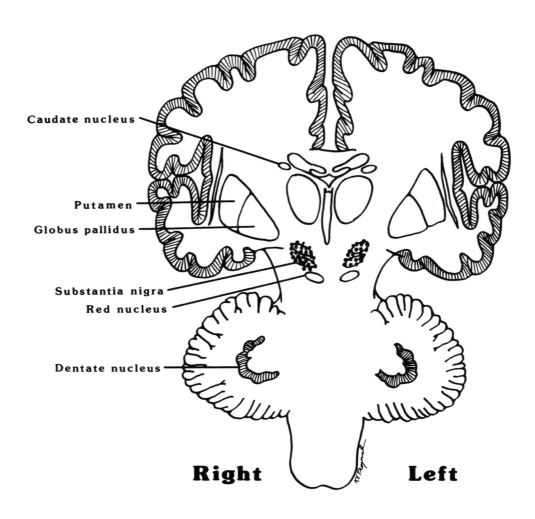

Caudate nucleus

Putamen

Globus pallidus

Substantia nigra
Red nucleus

Dentate nucleus

Right　　　**Left**

Impressions Hypokinetic dysarthria as a sign of Parkinson's disease.

Discussion In 1817 James Parkinson first described the clinical syndrome that now bears his name. Sometimes referred to as *paralysis agitans* as well, this disease most often afflicts persons in their fifth and sixth decades of life. It is a chronic, slowly progressive disorder ascribed to degeneration of dopamine-rich cells and tracts of the basal ganglia and, in particular, substantia nigra. The precipitating cause is as yet unknown.

The classic clinical portrait includes: (1) unremitting to-and-fro rest tremors of the head, (2) rest tremor of the thumb, index finger, and wrist of one or both hands, called *pill-rolling tremor*, and (3) limitations in the range (hypokinesia) and variable shifts in the speed (hastening) of movement of virtually all body parts. The latter conditions precipitate other signs of the disease, such as stooped posture, slow-shuffling gait, with intermittent and uncontrollable tendencies to increase the pace in a trotlike manner (festination), masklike facial expression, and dysarthria.

The tremors, hastening phenomena, and festinating gait may be attributed to disturbances in the inhibitory functions of the extrapyramidal system. Reduced range of movement is largely due to problems with reciprocal contractions of opposing muscle pairs as well as widespread muscle hypertonicity (rigidity).

The speech disturbances of Parkinson's disease generally result from reductions and limitations of movement and hastening phenomena of the speech musculature, hence the term *hypokinetic dysarthria*. The most prominent dysarthric features include short rushes of speech; harsh-breathy and monopitch, monoloud phonation; and imprecise, rapid labial and lingual alternate motion rates.

Dopamine replacement therapy is frequently the treatment of choice in Parkinson's disease. The dysarthria may respond to medical and speech therapy.

11-Year-Old Female with History of Seizures and Speech Disturbance

History   This 11-year-old female has a significant history for a partial seizure disorder with secondary generalization and migraine headaches, which have been managed successfully with various medications. She has also experienced periods of increased somnolence, from which she is readily aroused and immediately attentive.

Her father noted that following her hospitalization for what was described as pneumonia, she showed progressive deterioration in speech. Additionally, sleepiness increased enough to cause her to fall asleep at a basketball game. Primidone (Mysoline), which she had been taking for seizure control, was discontinued; the family, however, did not notice improvement in speech. Recently, family members had observed that her eyelids are drooped and that she complained of occasional choking on liquids.

Examination   Examination was remarkable for bilateral ptosis and facial paresis, with the upper face being more paretic than the lower. Mild wrist extensor weakness and areflexia of the upper extremities with normal deep tendon reflexes in the lower extremities were observed. Denervation was not apparent on EMG; nerve conduction studies were normal. Thyroxin level and other screening chemistries were within normal limits.

Lip seal and strength were reduced. The mandible was at the midline without compromise in strength on elevation or depression. The soft palate was symmetrical at rest, while during phonation, posterior-superior movement was moderately to severely reduced. Tongue protrusion was symmetrical and to the midline, but strength was mildly reduced with resistance.

Moderate to severe hypernasality with nasal emission and compensatory depression of the nasal ala were evident. Oral manometric study could not be completed due to an incomplete and weak bilabial seal.

Oral alternate and sequential motion (diadochokinetic) rates were mildly irregular. Articulatory precision in contextual speech was grossly within normal limits. Protracted effortful speaking, however, resulted in progressive deterioration of intelligibility.

Voice quality was marked by a mild, gurgly (wet) hoarseness. Rigid indirect fiberoptic laryngoscopy revealed incomplete vocal cord approximation. Affectively, the patient was appropriate, although the bilateral facial paresis and ptosis gave the impression that she was depressed. An edrophonium chloride (Tensilon) test revealed rapid improvement in motor function of the velopharynx, lip, tongue, and facial muscles.

29

Salient symptoms/signs	Test results	Impressions

This worksheet is to be used for recording relevant diagnostic observations. This step should be completed prior to turning to the Impressions. No figure for this case.

Impressions   Flaccid dysarthria secondary to myoneuropathy: Myasthenia gravis.

Discussion   *Myasthenia gravis* is characterized by abnormally rapid fatigue of muscle contractions. With rest, however, potential is improved. This condition is thought to be due to impairment of the release or uptake of acetylcholine at the myoneural junctions of the peripheral nervous system. Although various and random muscle groups may be affected throughout the body, the disease most often affects muscles of the speech mechanism.

The diagnosis of this disorder is confirmed by a positive Tensilon test. Using this clinical-drug procedure, the examiner should witness rapid improvement in the motor functioning of involved musculature. This was observed in our case, whose hypernasality and articulatory imprecision were reduced following administration of this drug. It should be noted that patients may develop mild bradycardia and sweating as side effects to this procedure.

When improvements are noted with Tensilon, the patient is frequently placed on pyridostigmine bromide (Mestinon), a drug that inhibits destruction of acetylcholine, thereby permitting freer transmission of nerve impulses across the myoneural junction. This drug proved beneficial for our patient. However, abdominal cramps, nausea, and vomiting are sometimes reported as side effects of Mestinon.

It is important to note that speech deteriorates with protracted effort and exertion in this type of neuromuscular disease; dysarthric signs are therefore rather inconsistent. Dysarthrias caused by a muscle disease (myopathy) or damage to a peripheral nerve (neuropathy), however, are relatively constant in their salient features.

79-Year-Old Male with Emotional Lability and Speech Disturbance

History

A 79-year-old retired male farmer experienced a severe dizzy spell that lasted several days. During this time he complained of a severe headache and exhibited virtually unintelligible speech. He remained in bed for a period of three months because of episodes of light-headedness and vertigo when attempting to get up. His speech gradually improved during this time of bed rest and he did not complain of limb weakness or swallowing difficulties.

For the past six months he has been using a cane for walking, without which he feels unsteady on his feet and tends to fall to the left. Since this time his speech has become progressively worse, which prompted medical and speech evaluations.

Examination

The left arm was resistive to passive movement and hyperreflexive. Gait was unsteady and slow. A Babinski sign was observed on the left.

The lower two-thirds of the face lacked emotional expression, though automatic or reactive movements of the facial muscles were observable. Facial contour and landmarks, such as the nasolabial folds, were unaffected. Circumoral and adjacent facial musculature movements during acts of lip pursing, smiling and laughing were bilaterally slow-labored, reduced in range and strength of contraction, and imprecise.

No signs of atrophy or fasciculations of the tongue were noted; however, nonspeech and speech movements were limited in range, weak, slow-labored, and imprecise. Resistance to passive movement was marked.

At rest, the velum was not remarkable. During vowel prolongation its movements were symmetrical, but limited in range. Isolated and connected speech were marked by hypernasal resonance and nasal snorting. Gag reflex was moderately hyperactive. Voice was perceived as strained in quality and coughing was perceived as weak.

Although unprovoked, the patient occasionally laughed and cried throughout testing, and appeared to be unable to control such emotional incontinence.

Receptive and expressive language skills were normal. Consonant and vowel productions during all speaking and oral alternate and sequential motion rate tasks were imprecise and slow-labored. Resonance was hypernasal, accompanied by episodes of nasal air escape; nasal regurgitation of liquids was also noted. Voice was strained-strangled in quality, with intermittent periods of phonatory arrest.

Worksheet

Salient symptoms/signs	Test results	Impressions

This worksheet is to be used for recording relevant diagnostic observations. The blank illustration is to be used for identifying and sketching the suspected site of lesion(s). These steps should be completed prior to turning to the Impressions and illustrated site of lesion.

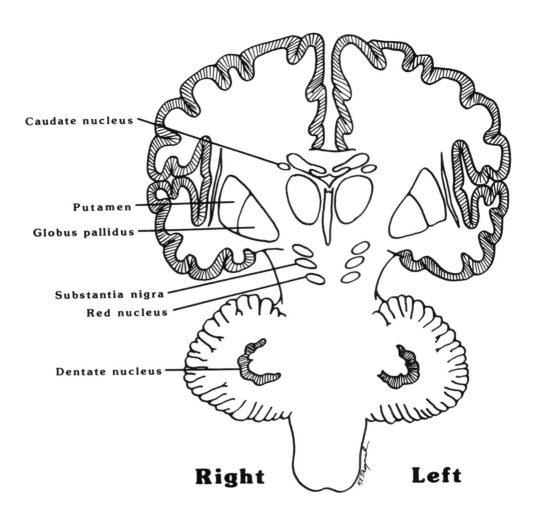

Caudate nucleus

Putamen

Globus pallidus

Substantia nigra

Red nucleus

Dentate nucleus

Right   **Left**

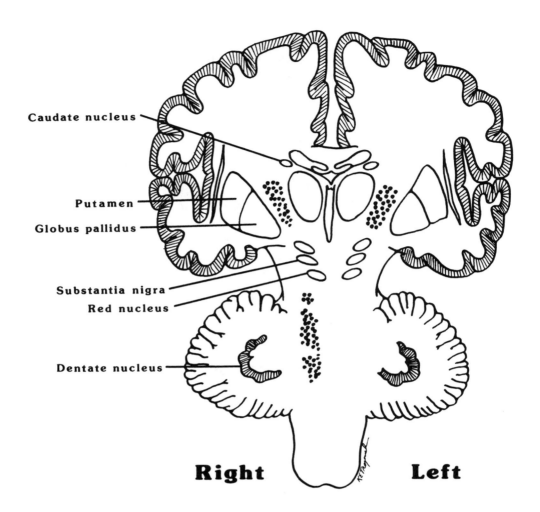

Caudate nucleus

Putamen

Globus pallidus

Substantia nigra
Red nucleus

Dentate nucleus

Right   **Left**

Impressions   Spastic dysarthria with unilateral left hemiparesis.

Discussion   The bilateral speech and unilateral limb neuromuscular abnormalities in this case are due, respectively, to bilateral corticobulbar and unilateral right corticospinal tract damage. CT scan suggested multiple lacunar strokes.

The term *pseudobulbar palsy* is used to differentiate the signs of bilateral involvement of the corticobulbar tract fibers that lead to and synapse with motor nuclei of the Vth, VIIth, IXth, Xth, XIth, and XIIth cranial nerves from the signs of lower motor neuron involvement including the nuclei themselves (bulbar palsy); hence the term *pseudobulbar.*

Muscles of the jaw, face, palate, pharynx, tongue, and larynx can be weak and variably immobile in either condition, and cause significant articulatory, resonatory, and phonatory impairments. However, whereas spastic muscles have increased tone, are resistive to passive movement, are marked by spasms, are hyperreflexic, and are not characterized by wasting or atrophy, flaccid muscles have decreased tone, yield to passive movement, are marked by flabbiness, are hyporeflexic, and are characterized by atrophy and fasciculations.

Being familiar with, and noting, these differences during testing is indispensable to reaching an accurate diagnosis. Further, patients with pseudobulbar palsy occasionally exhibit emotional lability—unprovoked crying and laughing—due to damage to pathways that normally inhibit or modulate these behaviors.

16-Year-Old Male with a History of Substance Abuse, Learning Disability, and Closed Head Injury

History

The patient is a 16-year-old, right-handed male with a history of substance abuse including alcohol, cocaine, crack (cocaine), heroin, and "angel dust" and a severe learning disability for which he had been receiving special education services. He was admitted to the ER by ambulance after falling off the back of a moving pick-up truck. On examination, his pupils were fixed and dilated and he was nonresponsive. Emergency CT scan showed a depressed right temporo-parietal skull fracture and an epidural hematoma with a moderate degree of mass effect and shift from right to left. A craniotomy was performed and the hematoma was successfully evacuated. The patient, however, remained in a comatose, but medically stable state for seven weeks. An EEG obtained during that period showed moderate bihemispheric slowing. He was independently breathing, not requiring ventilation. Repeat CT scan showed areas of mixed attenuation within the left frontal lobe at the level of the lateral ventricles; this study was otherwise normal. On awakening from coma, the patient was placed on phenytoin sodium (Dilantin) for seizure prophylaxis and discharged to the head injury unit. Multidisciplinary evaluations were conducted during the course of his stay.

Examination

General findings included (1) right hemiplegia with mildly wide-based gait, (2) decreased and irregular alternate motion rates of all four limbs, (3) discoordinated movements of the arms and legs, (4) decreased strength in the right arm and leg, (5) severe ataxia, and (6) mildly impaired aerobic capacity and endurance. Neuropsychologic examination showed severe impairment in the areas of (1) verbal memory, (2) spelling, (3) written language, (4) vocabulary, (5) judgment, (6) spatial orientation, (7) reaction time, and (8) arithmetic skills. He also had vegetative signs of severe depression and denial. His attention was poor. Neurocognitive/language evaluation revealed auditory and reading comprehension severe impairment, aberrant sentence content (semantics) and structure in connected discourse, and poor concrete thought, and pragmatic use of language.

Motor speech testing illustrated moderately slowed and irregularly timed dysdiadochokinesias of the tongue, lips, and jaw. Discoordinated fine and gross force of these muscles was evident in all vectors of movement. Articulation was imprecise; prosody disturbed by loudness outbursts and excess and equal stress. Resonance balance and vocal quality were normal; orofacial and muscle strength and gross anatomy were unaffected.

Worksheet

Salient symptoms/signs	Test results	Impressions

This worksheet is to be used for recording relevant diagnostic observations. The blank illustration is to be used for identifying and sketching the suspected site of lesion(s). These steps should be completed prior to turning to the Impressions and illustrated site of lesion.

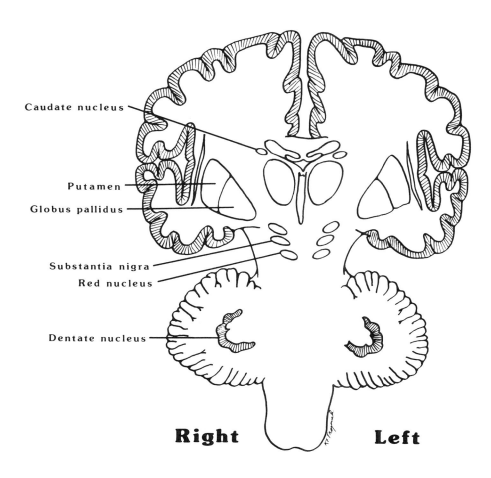

Caudate nucleus

Putamen

Globus pallidus

Substantia nigra

Red nucleus

Dentate nucleus

Right   **Left**

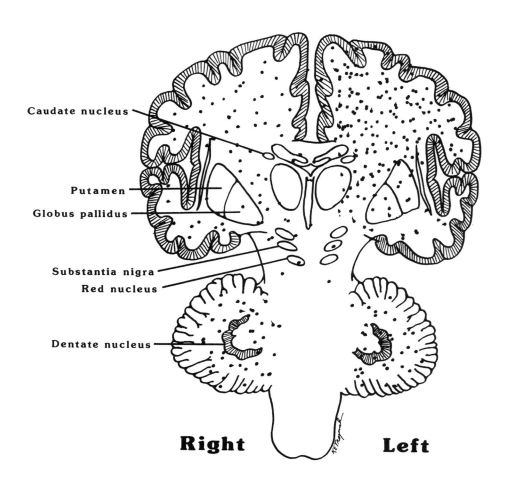

Caudate nucleus

Putamen

Globus pallidus

Substantia nigra

Red nucleus

Dentate nucleus

Right　　　　　　**Left**

Impressions   Confused language with associated neurocognitive impairment; ataxic dysarthria subsequent to closed head injury in a patient with a history of substance abuse and learning disability.

Discussion   The patient exhibited patterns of neuropsychological and neurolinguistic deficits typical of diffuse closed head injury. Because of impaired judgment that frequently accompanies patients with a learning disability and those who are substance abusers, it is probable that his premorbid status put him at great risk for a closed head injury.

Although neuroimaging studies showed a left cerebral hemisphere focus, the neurocognitive and language findings pointed to more widespread central nervous system damage caused by possibly coup-contra-coup injury and diffuse axonal shear. The wide-based, unbalanced gait, dysdiadochokinesia, articulatory discoordination, and prosodic breakdowns were suggestive of cerebellar dysfunction.

In conjunction with an intensive residential multidisciplinary treatment program, intervention stressed improvement of attention; memory through use of daily journals, checklists, and so on; cognitive and language skills through individual and group therapy programs; motor speech function through oral neuromotor speech stimulation and prosodic exercises; general motor behaviors through physical therapy; and vocational awareness through group and individual guidance sessions. Given his history and severity of his current injury, the prognosis for functional independence was fair.

Impressions   Severe speech/oral apraxia, with comparable aphasia secondary to metastatic adeno-carcinoma.

Discussion   The CT scan suggested a lesion in the left temporal lobe with considerable edema. At surgery this was confirmed, with the left operculum and posterior temporal and anterior parietal lobe areas showing edema.

   The patient's aphasia could adequately be accounted for by the temporal lobe lesion and posterior edema, while the swelling in the area of the left operculum was thought to account for the speech apraxia.

   Preservation of rather simple comprehension abilities, including knowledge of nonverbal gesture, is not atypical in dense language disorders. On a linguistic hierarchy, knowledge of gestures, without the influence of either an auditory or visual cue, is usually rather low.

   The severity of this patient's impairment makes differentiating apraxia from aphasia difficult. However, her inability to retain water in her mouth in the absence of oral neuromuscular involvement, suggests that she had difficulty planning the sequences of movement necessary to move the water posteriorly. Her limited verbal output, of course, could have represented both the aphasia and apraxia of speech. There were no instances, however, of jargon, neologistic distortion, or perseveration noted in her verbal output.

   Approximately one week following excision of the tumor, the patient's communicative signs improved to the point where she demonstrated only a moderate oral or speech dyspraxia and comparable dysphasia. Radiation, speech, physical, and occupational therapy were initiated and continued on an outpatient basis. Seizure medications were continued as a precautionary measure. She was discharged in the care of her internist and oncologist. Three months after discharge from hospital, she died.

72-Year-Old Male with a History of Respiratory Arrest, Coma

History   The patient is a 72-year-old, right-handed male with a history of a spontaneous respiratory arrest associated with a myocardial infarction and coma eleven years before being seen. He also had work-related chronic obstructive pulmonary disease (COPD) as formerly a painter for an automobile manufacturer. Admitted to the general medicine service with a ten-day history of fever, chills, reduced oral intake, and weakness, the patient was found to have pneumonia and congestive heart failure, with exacerbation of his COPD. His condition gradually improved with antibiotic therapies. During the course of his hospitalization, however, there were questions raised about his communicative-cognitive status. He was, therefore, referred for evaluation.

Examination   The patient was awake, alert, well-oriented to events and surroundings. He emphatically denied changes in either speech or language and stated that his memory was "as good as ever." He did complain of chronic tingling of the right arm since his respiratory arrest eleven years earlier; other than his resolving weakness secondary to current hospitalization, he had no other complaints.

With the exception of exaggerated physiologic head tremor, the motor speech examination was within normal limits. Expressive language was grammatically and generally semantically sound, although rather concrete. Visual fields were normal on both single and double simultaneous stimulation testing. He had no difficulty following one-step through two-step complex verbal commands, obtaining information from simple to complex sentences presented visually, performing simple mental computation, or writing simple words or sentences to dictation. When challenged with more complex computation, he asked "Does plus mean add or take away?" He had difficulty determining the relationships between paired common related objects. He stated there were 48 weeks in a year. Visual perceptual signs were evident on a task requiring replication of a three-dimensional cube. He was unable to recall four common, but unrelated nouns within a three-minute period.

Neuropsychological testing revealed mild right-left confusion, impaired visual perceptual/motor skills, a verbal IQ of 73, performance IQ of 78, and a full scale IQ of 74. He was anosagnostic (unaware, unappreciative) regarding any of the signs delineated on speech pathology or neuropsychology evaluations.

MRI of the brain showed generalized cerebral atrophy and enlarged ventricles.

Salient symptoms/signs	Test results	Impressions

This worksheet is to be used for recording relevant diagnostic observations. The blank illustration is to be used for identifying and sketching the suspected site of lesion(s). These steps should be completed prior to turning to the Impressions and illustrated site of lesion.

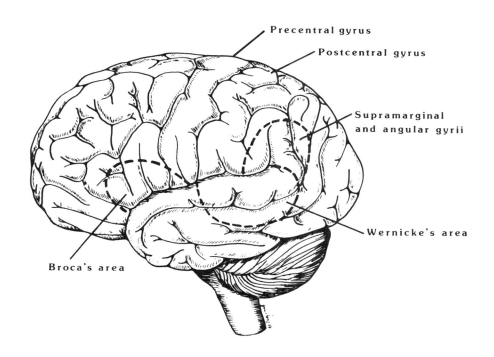

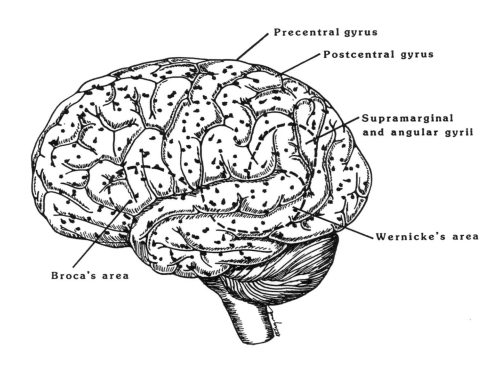

Precentral gyrus

Postcentral gyrus

Supramarginal
and angular gyrii

Wernicke's area

Broca's area

Impressions   Generalized intellectual impairment (dementia) status post respiratory arrest: anoxic encephalopathy.

Discussion   Overall, the patient's neurocommunicative/cognitive deficits were judged mild to moderate in degree and were believed to be caused by sequelae of his cardiac arrest and coma, and associated neurodegenerative changes supported by the clinical and neuroimaging findings. Because the arrest had occurred eleven years before the hospitalization leading to evaluation, it appeared that the patient had been doing quite well in view of the deficits demonstrated on examination. His wife had been managing the checkbook and paying the bills; he had chosen not to work around machinery or drive—insightful decisions for a patient with dementia. He was determined not to be a candidate for cognitive therapy and has, therefore, to be seen on an as-needed basis.

31-Year-Old Male with Closed Head Injury, Hypertonicity, and Speech Disturbance

History This 31-year-old male was involved in a car accident in which he was knocked unconscious. His Glasgow Coma Scale score at the scene of the accident was 6, and he was immediately rushed to the trauma center.

On admission, he was in a comatose state. He had fractures of the fifth through twelfth thoracic ribs on the left side. Associated diminution of breath sounds, and reduction of resonance to percussion testing in the left lower lung field were also noted.

A chest tube was inserted to assist ventilation. Peritoneal lavage was negative. Cervical spine x-rays were also negative. A small right frontal contusion was detected clinically and on CT scan. Intracranial pressure was monitored, and increased readings were evident. He was treated with phenytoin sodium (Dilantin) and mannitol.

Three days after admission he developed a left lower lobe pneumonia with positive cultures for hemophilus influenza and streptococcus fecalis. These were treated with gentamicin sulfate and ampicillin. Within one week the pneumonia was resolved. CT scans performed one month later revealed no dramatic findings or treatable lesion sites.

A nasogastric tube was inserted to aid in maintaining nourishment, and a tracheostomy was performed to prevent further pulmonary infections. The patient remained in a semicomatose state for seven months, during which complete assessments were not feasible. Following this state, when his level of consciousness had improved, an extensive examination was conducted.

Examination The following test data were collected: (1) vital signs normal; (2) pupils equal, round, and reactive to light; (3) pharynx clear; (4) tracheostomy tube was removed as breathing appeared improved over prearousal levels; (5) supple neck with no bruits; (6) persistent crackles and diminished breath sounds in left lung; (7) quadriparesis, more severe on the right side; (8) marked hyperactivity of knee and ankle jerks; (9) spasticity of all four extremities; (10) bilateral Babinski signs; (11) painful stimuli are appreciated, but pinprick and proprioceptive testing revealed moderate impairments in the lower limbs; (12) assistance is needed to move from a supine to sitting position; (13) markedly reduced breath support for speech; (14) moderate weakness of the tongue; (15) bilateral paresis of the lower two-thirds of the facies; (16) bilateral velopharyngeal paralysis, with associated atrophy and absent gag reflex; (17) hypernasality and nasal snorting; (18) breathy dysphonia with phrases of one to two words, at best; (19) laryngologic exam revealed bilateral vocal cord paralysis in the paramedian position; (20) markedly slow-labored rate of speech, and lingual and labial diadochokinetic rates; (21) mildly impaired auditory discrimination, retention span, and receptive vocabulary; (22) mild word-finding errors; (23) marked articulatory imprecision; and (24) monopitch and monoloud vocal patterns.

CT scans, EEG, chest x-rays, and sputum cultures were normal. Signs of emotional lability, characterized by short burst of anger, frustration, and withdrawal, were evident.

Worksheet

Salient symptoms/signs	Test results	Impressions

This worksheet is to be used for recording relevant diagnostic observations. The blank illustration is to be used for identifying and sketching the suspected site of lesion(s). These steps should be completed prior to turning to the Impressions and illustrated site of lesion.

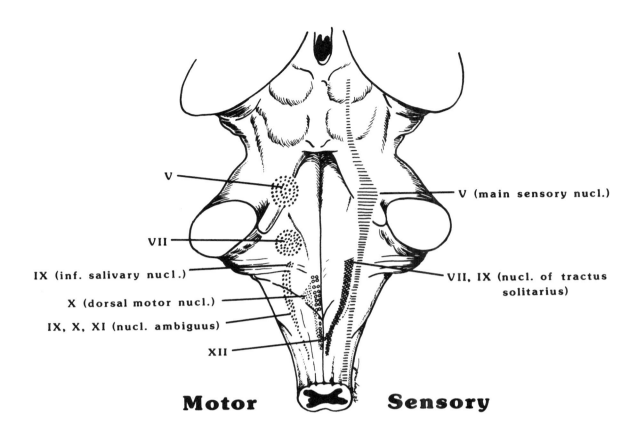

V

V (main sensory nucl.)

VII

IX (inf. salivary nucl.)

X (dorsal motor nucl.)

IX, X, XI (nucl. ambiguus)

XII

VII, IX (nucl. of tractus
solitarius)

Motor **Sensory**

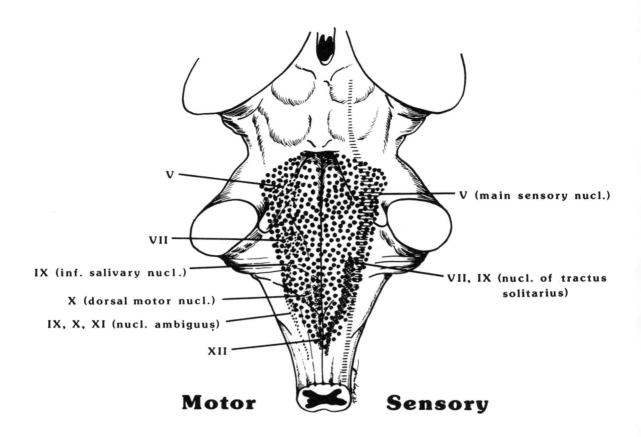

V

V (main sensory nucl.)

VII

IX (inf. salivary nucl.)

X (dorsal motor nucl.)

IX, X, XI (nucl. ambiguus)

XII

VII, IX (nucl. of tractus solitarius)

Motor   **Sensory**

Impressions Mixed spastic-flaccid dysarthria caused by closed head injury.

Discussion A closed head injury is one in which the skull is only minimally fractured or bruised. The degree of impact varies from accident to accident, as do the resultant clinical profiles.

Mild injuries do not usually cause lasting neurologic changes or significant clinical findings. On occasion, a brief loss of consciousness and retrograde amnesia occur.

Moderate injuries may result in longer periods of unconsciousness, and various neurologic symptoms and signs. Swelling and contusions of intracranial tissue, including the brain and brainstem, are not uncommon.

Severe injuries usually result in prolonged unconsciousness and a multitude of abnormal clinical and laboratory neurologic test findings.

Our patient had a severe closed head injury, with an associated severe symptom complex. His prolonged state of unconsciousness indicates, as in most cases like this, severe damage to the brainstem. His clinical portrait substantiates this conclusion; that is, his symptoms and signs are suggestive of brainstem injury.

Spastic quadriparesis with associated paresis, hypertonicity, and exaggerated stretch reflexes are manifestations of bilateral pyramidal system (corticospinal tract) impairment; paresis, and hypertonicity of the tongue and facies are signs of bilateral pyramidal system (corticobulbar tract) involvement. Note that facial paralysis in this case is different from the facial paralysis caused by VIIth cranial nerve (peripheral nervous system) involvement. In the latter, the muscles of the entire side of the face are affected: forehead, orbit, cheek, lips, and chin. Such tissue will be hypotonic (flaccid) and may atrophy on the same side(s) as that of the nerve damage. In the former (our) case, only the lower two-thirds (below the orbits) of the face is involved on the side(s) opposite the lesion site(s). The musculature is generally hypertonic, and no atrophy occurs. The velopharyngeal and laryngeal signs are indicative of Xth cranial nerve damage. This nerve (vagus) innervates the larynx and pharynx. When it is damaged the innervated musculature becomes weak, dystrophic and hypoactive.

Collectively, the tongue, face, and lip signs (spastic), and the velopharyngeal and laryngeal signs (flaccid) have given this patient a severe form of mixed dysarthria. His poor breath support and mild language impairment compound his communicative disability. His emotional lability is not uncommon for those with a serious head injury. Headache, memory deficits, poor attention span, and personality shifts are also associated with head injury.

The patient underwent physical, occupational, and speech-language therapy. He is confined to a wheelchair, but improved in the use of his hands for self-help needs. Speech-language intervention focused on facilitating: (1) auditory language comprehension; (2) expressive language; and (3) improvements in the tone, strength, speed, and control of the tongue musculature in order to increase articulatory intelligibility.

Laryngologic consultations prompted recommendation for Teflon® injection of one vocal cord to improve phonation. Prosthodontic consultations have led to the construction of a palatal lift device to aid in velopharyngeal closure for reduction of hypernasality.

57-Year-Old Male with Positive Stroke History and Speech Disturbance

History

This 57-year-old man was admitted to hospital after he collapsed at work. His wife informed the admitting nurse that her husband had a history of two strokes, one 10 years and another just eight months prior to this incident. They were thought to be embolic in origin, following acute myocardial infarction and atrial fibrillation, respectively.

His first stroke resulted in a short clinical course. Initially he exhibited a moderate degree of left hemiparesis with involvement of the lower two-thirds of the left face and entire left half of the tongue. The resultant gait and motor speech difficulties lasted only a week. Within one month, the patient was able to return to work.

Approximately nine years passed before the patient's second stroke that resulted in right hemiparesis and involvement of the lower two-thirds of the face and half of the tongue on the right. Gait and motor speech difficulties were mild to moderate in degree and short-lived. Once again, within four to six weeks the patient returned fulltime to work.

There were no impending stroke signs or symptoms prior to his collapse on the loading dock. The patient seemed to be doing quite well. His blood pressure, pulse rate, and overall heart condition were being monitored by his family physician on a regular basis, and he had been taking anticoagulants since his last stroke.

Examination

The patient, 5'10" tall and 146 lbs, was alert and cooperative, and appeared to comprehend verbal instructions. Eyes, ears, nose, and throat were normal. Pupils were equal, round, and reactive to light, with normal fundoscopic findings. Visual field defects could not be determined.

Bruits were not heard in either carotid. Cardiac examination and electrocardiogram revealed severe auricular fibrillation; heartbeat was abnormal and variable with regard to rate, rhythm, and intensity. The pulse was slow, with irregularly long diastolic pauses; blood pressure was 185/115. Right hemiparesis was evident, with concommitant brisk deep tendon and Babinski signs on that side.

There was mild weakness of the lower two-thirds of the face on the right with moderately good bilateral lip activities upon request. The tongue deviated to the right upon protrusion, was weak and mildly slow in its movements. No other motor, sensory, reflex or coordinative abnormalities were noted.

Cerebrospinal fluid analysis and skull x-ray proved normal. Cerebral angiography revealed an obstruction in the ascending frontal branch of the middle cerebral artery. CT scan revealed an infarct in the infero-lateral-posterior region of the left frontal lobe.

Test of oral praxis showed significant deficits in volitional non-speech movements of the lips, tongue, and jaw musculature; automatic or reactive adjustments of these same structures were preserved. Oral alternate and sequential motion rates were markedly imprecise and slow. Sound and syllable reversals and transpositions were apparent.

Spontaneous speech was characterized by articulatory groping, false starts, abnormal prolongations within and between words, repetitions of individual sounds, and multiple yet variable articulation errors. Words of increasing length provoked more of these articulatory breakdowns. Initiating speech, especially with words of phonetic complexity, was particularly difficult. Prompts by the examiner were only marginally helpful. Great frustration seemed to accompany all volitional speech efforts.

Auditory, visual and reading comprehension remained intact. Writing and penmanship skills were good with the nonpreferred hand, both spontaneously and to dictation. Complex language tasks, requiring non-verbal responses, were performed accurately.

Worksheet

Salient symptoms/signs	Test results	Impressions

This worksheet is to be used for recording relevant diagnostic observations. The blank illustration is to be used for identifying and sketching the suspected site of lesion(s). These steps should be completed prior to turning to the Impressions and illustrated site of lesion.

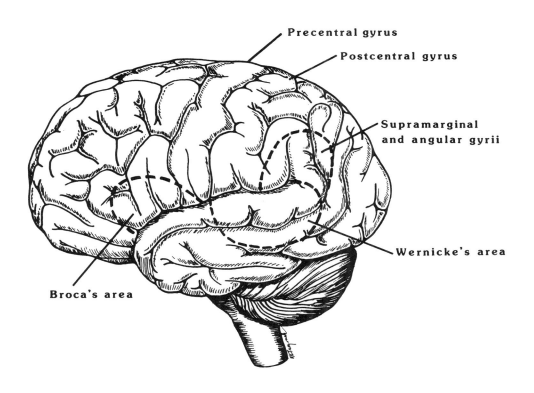

Precentral gyrus

Postcentral gyrus

Supramarginal
and angular gyrii

Wernicke's area

Broca's area

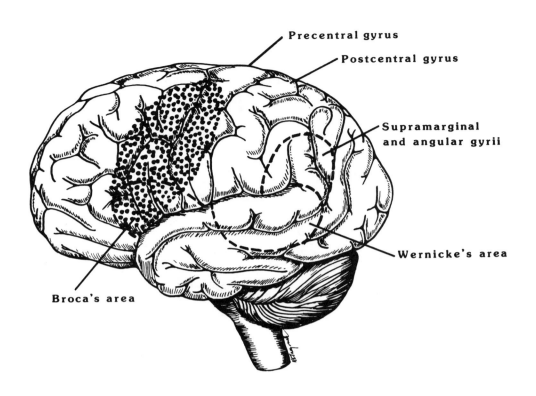

Precentral gyrus

Postcentral gyrus

Supramarginal
and angular gyrii

Wernicke's area

Broca's area

Impressions   Speech apraxia secondary to embolic stroke.

Discussion   Cerebral infarction is the cause of nearly all strokes except those due to hemorrhage. A cerebral infarct is defined as an area of brain in which the blood flow has fallen below the critical level necessary to maintain the viability of the tissue.

Cerebral blood vessels may be occluded by emboli that arise elsewhere (e.g., the heart or the carotid artery) or by thrombi that occur in situ. Embolic infarction is often preceded by transient ischemic attacks while thrombolic infarctions are not. In completed strokes the neurological deficits last more than 24 hours and may be permanent. The nature and extent of the deficit depend upon the area of brain and arterial territory involved.

Cerebral hemorrhage most often occurs in the setting of long-standing hypertension. It can also be the result of a ruptured aneurysm or vascular malformation. Sudden severe headache followed by hemiplegia and progression to coma is a common mode of presentation. Smaller hematomas, of course, will result in proportionately larger deficit. Recognizing the various types of strokes is essential in planning the management of each patient.

Our patient's stroke was embolic in nature. The embolus originated from the heart and travelled via the left internal carotid artery to the middle cerebral artery and finally lodged in its ascending frontal branch, which supplies Broca's area.

The role of Broca's area in speech and language has been a hotly debated subject for many years. Most researchers agree, however, that it aids in syllable and word sequencing; in programming the elemental postures of the articulatory mechanism during speech production; and in maintaining speech rhythm and coordinated sound transitions.

Our patient's speech apraxia without aphasia helps to confirm the existence of a separate system that subserves motor speech programming. Although uncommon, this system can be selectively impaired.

The right hemiparesis and associated motor and sensory disturbances in our patient implicate the left pyramidal system, including both corticobulbar (face and tongue symptoms) and corticospinal (limb and trunk symptoms) tracts. Because the origin and course of this system is in neuroanatomic proximity to Broca's area, lesions of the frontal lobe frequently cause co-occurring apraxia/aphasia and contralateral hemiparesis.

The motor speech effects of the unilateral tongue and lip musculature involvement were judged to be minimal. Speech therapy included alternate and sequential motion rate tasks and contrastive stress drills. The prognosis remained guarded.

40-Year-Old Male with a Change in Voice

History This patient, a 40-year-old, right-handed male, was referred for further evaluation of phonatory/laryngologic function by an otolaryngologist whose earlier examination results read normal. The patient's medical history was noncontributory; as an athlete and football coach, he was in excellent health.

The patient complained of a change in voice characterized by hoarseness and "pitch breaks," which had begun during the basketball season. From onset of the symptoms, his voice had never returned to normal, although on occasion, it had improved. Overall, however, there had been slight progression of the symptoms noticed mostly by his wife and friends. He had noted that his voice consistently worsened when anxious and stressed and improved when he was relaxed. There was no history of previous voice or speech problems; he had not experienced difficulty swallowing or breathing. His voice did not change after exercise or with ethanol. He denied changes in vision, handwriting, gait, or muscle strength. The family history was negative for a communication or movement disorder.

The patient was not taking prescription medication. There were no gastroesophageal symptoms. The patient denied depression or psycho-emotional discord. There were no language or cognitive complaints. His coaching career was both active and successful.

Examination Function for cranial nerves V (motor and sensory), VII, and IX through XII was clinically within normal limits. There were no pathologic reflexes. The structural integrity of the speech mechanism was sound for speech production. With the exception of the phonatory/laryngeal signs, the remainder of the motor speech examination result was well within normal limits.

Conversational speech was characterized by moderate/severe intermittent strained-strangled quality, harshness, and periodic fleeting cessation of phonation. Maximum phonation time averaged 20 seconds on vowel prolongation; there were no perceptual features of voice tremor. Rigid laryngo videostroboscopic examination showed periodic adductory occlusion of the vocal folds and supraglottic structures during prolongation of a neutral vowel. On occasion, facial grimacing occurred in synchrony with the perceived voice arrests. A brief trial of behavioral voice therapy did not render improvement in voice quality.

Language and cognitive functions were well within normal limits. With the exception of the phonatory signs, subsequent neurologic evaluation also proved normal.

Salient symptoms/signs	Test results	Impressions

This worksheet is to be used for recording relevant diagnostic observations. The blank illustration is to be used for identifying and sketching the suspected site of lesion(s). These steps should be completed prior to turning to the Impressions and illustrated site of lesion.

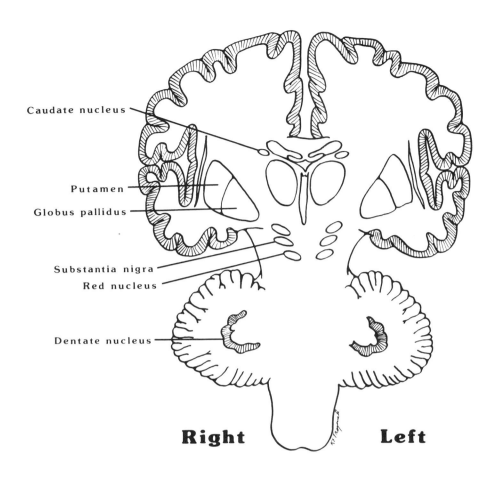

Caudate nucleus

Putamen

Globus pallidus

Substantia nigra

Red nucleus

Dentate nucleus

Right   **Left**

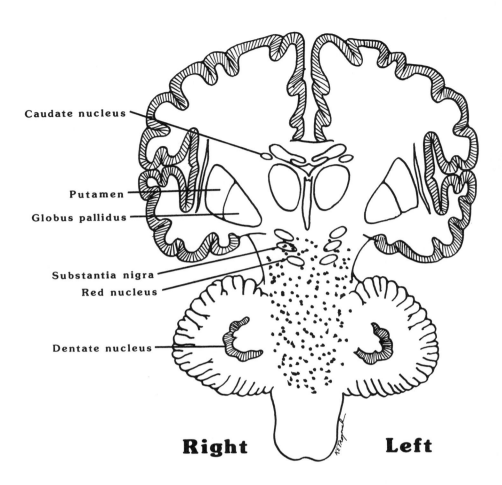

Caudate nucleus

Putamen

Globus pallidus

Substantia nigra

Red nucleus

Dentate nucleus

Right   **Left**

Impressions   Moderate/severe spasmodic dysphonia of the adductor type; focal laryngeal dystonia.

Discussion   Laryngospasm (voice arrest), occurs in normal physiological activities, including defecation, micturition, and lifting. It can be also manifested in pathologic conditions such as spasmodic dysphonia, which may represent a focal movement disorder including laryngeal dystonia, essential tremor, and, less frequently, psychopathology. Our patient exhibited strained quality, harshness, and laryngospasm consistent with this diagnosis.

Intermittent spasms, from hyperactive laryngeal function may occur with the vocal folds postured in adducted (closed) and/or abducted (open) positions. Abnormal contractions of the pharyngeal and orofacial musculature frequently co-occur with the phonatory signs.

In actuality, spasmodic dysphonia, as a focal laryngeal dystonia or a component of voice tremor, is a hyperkinetic dysarthria. However features of spasmodic dysphonia may also be present in other neurogenic disorders of speech such as spastic dysarthria. Spastic dysarthria, however, is characterized more by strained-strangled quality than by voice arrest, as well as other signs of motor speech involvement.

If the patient's history and clinical findings support a psychological etiology, then a period of behavioral therapy that may include direct voice therapy and psychotherapy is indicated. Although there are reports of effective behavioral therapy for spasmodic dysphonia, the prognosis for improvement with this mode of treatment is generally poor for all forms of the disorders.

Within the past few years, intramuscular laryngeal injections of botulinum toxin have evolved as the standard of treatment for spasmodic dysphonia. For patients with the adductor form of the disorder, injections are placed directly into the thyroarytenoid musculature. For the less common abductor form, injections are placed into the posterior cricoarytenoid musculature and, on occasion, cricothyroid muscles. The injections produce myoneural junction blockade, creating weakness in the treated muscles. Goals for the adductor form, then, are a reduction or elimination of the voice arrest with improved vocal quality. For the abductor form, the anticipated results include improved approximation of the vocal folds for voicing and phonation. Because sprouting of collateral nerve endings in treated muscles can cause spasms to recur, patients generally require repeated injections every 3 to 6 months. Now, there are only anecdotal reports concerning the long-term systemic effects of therapeutic botulinum toxin.

As illustrated, the site of lesion for the neurogenic form of spasmodic dysphonia is believed to be within the brainstem. Our patient elected to be followed rather than be currently considered for botulinum toxin therapy. He is, therefore, seen for re-evaluation on a regular basis.

8-Year-Old Female with Recurrent, Progressive Headaches, Motor Incoordination, and Speech Disturbances

History An 8-year-old girl awoke one morning with a severe headache and feelings of nausea and increased pressure in the back of her head. These symptoms disappeared within 24 hours, enabling her to return to school. Over the course of the next six months she experienced recurrent and progressively more severe episodes of headaches, nausea, and vomiting, which were intensified or precipitated by physical exercise. She also had progressive lethargy, vertigo, motor incoordination of gait and upper limb activities, and slurred speech.

Examination The patient was alert and cooperative during testing. Her use of language was generally comprehensive and age appropriate, although she did exhibit occasional lapses with respect to time and recent events.

Gait was unsteady and wide-based, and she swayed when standing upright with feet together with her eyes open as well as closed. Finger-to-nose and heel-to-shin tasks were mildly incoordinated and tremulous, bilaterally, and provoked vertigo and imbalance; tremors did not occur at rest. Alternate motion rates of the hands, feet, and speech musculature were moderately slow and irregular. Contextual speech was variably imprecise and slow and marked by fluctuations in vowel quality, prolongations of phonemes and word intervals, and periodically explosive stress patterns. Voice was harsh in quality and reduced in pitch and loudness control. CT scan revealed dilatation of the fourth ventricle and abnormal density in the lateral cerebellar lobes.

Worksheet

Salient symptoms/signs	Test results	Impressions

This worksheet is to be used for recording relevant diagnostic observations. The blank illustration is to be used for identifying and sketching the suspected site of lesion(s). These steps should be completed prior to turning to the Impressions and illustrated site of lesion.

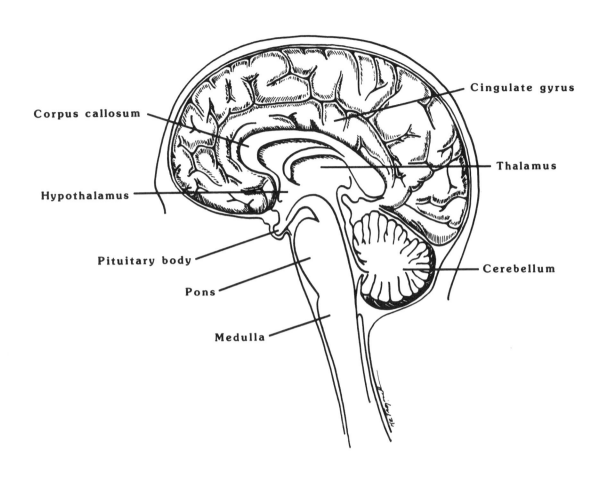

Corpus callosum

Hypothalamus

Pituitary body

Pons

Medulla

Cingulate gyrus

Thalamus

Cerebellum

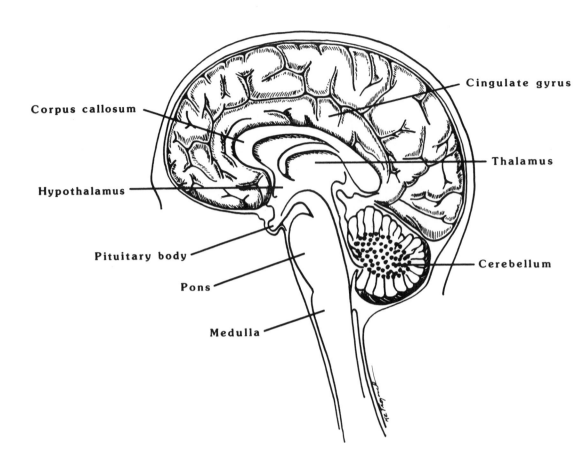

Corpus callosum

Hypothalamus

Pituitary body

Pons

Medulla

Cingulate gyrus

Thalamus

Cerebellum

Impressions   Ataxic dysarthria and quadriplegia.

Discussion   The signs and symptoms in this case point to a cerebellar lesion that proved to be, at surgery, an astrocytoma.

Approximately 60 percent of the primary brain tumors are astrocytomas that arise from astrocytes or glial cells. Astrocytomas may be relatively benign or highly malignant. The signs and symptoms depend upon the location and rate of growth. Typically symptoms begin insidiously and progress in a subacute fashion. Acute onset may occur with hemorrhage into the tumor. Symptoms and signs may be considered generalized or focal. Headaches, vomiting, and progressive deteriorations of alertness are examples of generalized symptoms and reflect raised intracranial pressure, hydrocephalus, and brain edema. Focal signs and symptoms are due to local destruction of brain tissue and may consist of aphasia, apraxia of speech, dysarthria, focal seizures, ataxia, cranial nerve palsies, and the like.

Unilateral cerebellar lesions cause ataxia of extremities on the same side, along with nystagmus, hypotonia, and frequently dysarthria. Midline lesions produce ataxia of the trunk, dysarthria, and gait ataxia. Extension into the fourth ventricle may result in obstructive hydrocephalus.

68-Year-Old Female with Progressive Memory Loss, Combativeness, Paranoia, and Language Disturbance

History This 68-year-old female, a former school teacher, was brought to the clinic by her spouse. He reported that, behaviorally, she had declined drastically over the past three years. Her primary care physician originally diagnosed her difficulties as "senility due to hardening of the arteries," for which blood-thinning drugs were prescribed along with a more balanced, low salt diet.

Over the past year, she had begun to exhibit: (1) progressive memory impairment, (2) catastrophic reactions to (even) innocuous stimuli, (3) coprolalic utterances, (4) violent and crude behaviors, (5) paranoia, (6) delusions, (7) aimless wandering, (8) nightmares, and (9) significant expressive and receptive language disturbances.

Examination The patient was uncooperative during testing. Frequently she exclaimed, "Get your goddam hands off of me!" as she attempted to leave the examination area. Simple commands and inquiries were typically met with no response or statements such as "What the hell do you care?" and "Leave me alone!" Extemporaneous speech was articulate and fluent, but semantically incoherent. Syntax, however, appeared relatively preserved.

On confrontation naming tasks, when the patient did respond without hostility, she was verbose, chose incorrect words, and responded incorrectly to many of the stimuli. She could point to and name various body parts fairly consistently, but mistakenly called a dog a cat, a car a truck and a knife a sword.

She could not pass the screening portions of various auditory and reading comprehension, picture vocabulary, or visual motor integration tests. Although she exhibited marked impairment naming common objects, she could gesture or pantomine their functions more often than not. Short- and long-term memory were severely limited.

General neurologic examination proved unremarkable; CT scan was normal. The oral speech mechanism was structurally within normal limits. No signs of weakness, paralysis, incoordination nor changes in the tone of the speech musculature were evident. Positron emission tomography (PET) scan revealed marked reduction of blood flow in the frontal-parietal-temporal zones of each cerebral hemisphere.

Salient symptoms/signs	Test results	Impressions

This worksheet is to be used for recording relevant diagnostic observations. The blank illustration is to be used for identifying and sketching the suspected site of lesion(s). These steps should be completed prior to turning to the Impressions and illustrated site of lesion.

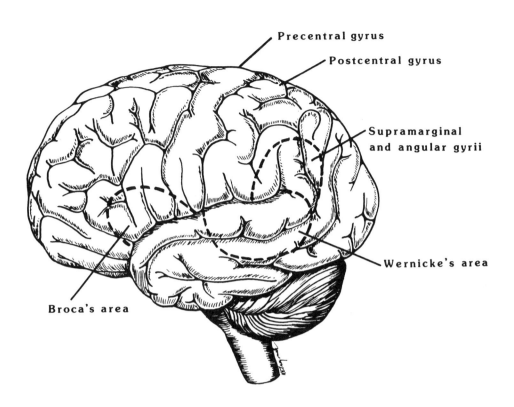

Precentral gyrus

Postcentral gyrus

Supramarginal
and angular gyrii

Wernicke's area

Broca's area

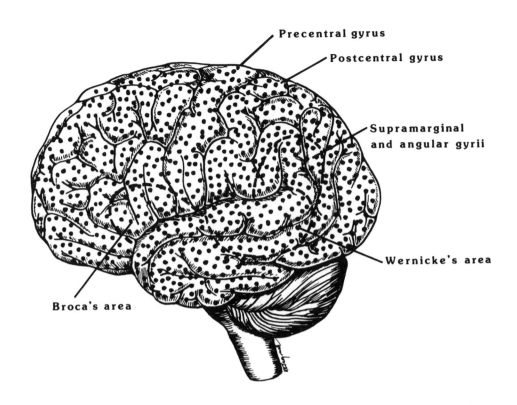

Precentral gyrus

Postcentral gyrus

Supramarginal and angular gyrii

Wernicke's area

Broca's area

Impressions   Generalized intellectual impairment, or dementia of the Alzheimer type.

Discussion   Alzheimer's disease (AD) was first recognized at the turn of this century by the German neurologist Alois Alzheimer. Originally it was considered a dementing condition of the elderly. We now know, however, that AD afflicts not only the elderly but those in their forties and fifties as well.

The neuropathologic changes underlying AD are not completely understood, nor are they completely predictable. What is known, however, is that within 3 to 10 years those with this dreadful disease will become severely demented and unable to care for themselves.

Although death does not result from the disease itself, in time these people die of complications that afflict incapacitated and bedridden individuals, such as urinary tract infections and pneumonia.

Unequivocal diagnosis of AD depends upon postmortem analysis of the brain or a brain biopsy. Virtually all those who exhibit the dementing symptoms, similar to those of the patient here presented, show, on autopsy, specific types of neuropathological abnormalities. These include neurofibrillary (paired helical) tangles and plaque formations particularly in the areas of the hippocampus, amygdala, and substantia innominata. Significant depletions in the neurotransmitters cholinesterase, somatostatin, and noradrenalin have also been detected in the brains of those with histories suggestive of AD.

Although AD affects multiple zones of the brain, only the gray matter is involved. In the dementias caused by illnesses other than AD, such as multiple infarcts, gray and white matter symptoms and signs are recognized. These may include higher cognitive, linguistic, and abstract reasoning disturbances as sequela to gray matter involvement, and sensorimotor impairments of speech or limb and trunk function due to white matter involvement.

It is worth noting that the dementia of AD usually follows a progressive steady course. The dementia that may result from multiple infarcts is also progressive, but in a stepwise fashion.

An arbitrary rating scale can be used to classify AD. In stage 1, the patient generally exhibits forgetfulness, mild memory deficits, difficulty with taking on new tasks, and depressed performance levels at work. Antidepressant drugs are sometimes prescribed in mild doses for patients in stage 1 of the disease.

In stage 2, mild to moderate psychiatric and behavioral problems emerge, as do speech and language disorders; the symptoms of stage 1 become even more pronounced, as well. Antipsychotic medications are frequently prescribed to decrease catastrophic reactions and agitated behavior patterns in stage 2.

Stage 3 is the final stage of AD. Here the patient has marked intellectual, cognitive, and behavioral dysfunctions. Taking care of oneself and communicating with one's environment is virtually impossible at this stage. At some point after progression to this level the patient will probably require institutionalization. Our patient might be said to be progressing into stage 3.

Whether the word-finding difficulties in the spontaneous speech of AD patients are manifestations of perceptual confusions (as in calling an outboard motor a fan), or breakdowns in complete awareness of the features that distinguish related items (as in calling a dog a cat) is not known. Our patient made both types of lexical errors.

In the second and third stages of AD, spontaneous speech becomes incoherent but fluent. Many patients with AD demonstrate good repetition of speech stimuli, even though various aspects of comprehension are significantly impaired. These signs are compatible with those seen in focal language disturbance, aphasia. Our patient did not echo speech stimuli; however, this may have been due to her uncooperativeness.

Whether gestural or pantomimic skills are disturbed in dementia of the Alzheimer type is still not fully understood. Our patient's gestural skills were relatively well preserved, despite significant problems finding associated words.

As patients with AD progress into stage 3, their behaviors may become dangerous to themselves, and those around them. Ultimately they become dependent upon others for their survival. Outside agencies such as the Alzheimer's Disease and Related Disorders Association (ADRDA) have been formed throughout the United States to assist families of patients stricken with AD. Support meetings, community education programs, and ongoing medical care are but a few of the functions of local ADRDA chapters.

Medical, speech-language, social work, and other professional practitioners and volunteers work closely to provide the best care for the patient with AD. Our patient received such care.

83-Year-Old Male with Acute Onset of Facial Weakness and Change in Speech

History This 83-year-old man described a history in which some thirteen years before being seen, he experienced a sharp sensation in his eyes while driving his automobile and subsequent generalized weakness of his face with a change in speech. Since onset, the symptoms had gradually progressed, but had remained stable for the previous 3 to 4 years. He maintained that his speech was generally understood; he had no difficulty swallowing, but had experienced occasional nasopharyngeal reflux. He had no breathing difficulty, changes in handwriting, or gait. There were no language or cognitive complaints. He denied change in muscle strength or bulk; there had been no cramping. A tensilon challenge and subsequent Mestinon trial for myasthenia by his internist proved equivocal in improving his condition. The patient was seen by a neurologist, who recommended an EMG and possible muscle biopsy, both of which the patient refused.

Examination On examination, the patient was awake, alert, and attentive. He had complete bilateral facial paralysis. The right eye was closed; the left eye was kept open with tape. He was unable to blink. To facilitate speech, he used the thumb of his right hand to approximate the mandible to the maxilla. He indicated also that he used this posture for feeding (chewing). He was unable to approximate the mandible to the maxilla otherwise. The soft palate was symmetrical at rest. A pharyngeal reflex was not elicited and posterior superior movement of the soft palate was either absent or showed equivocal movement. Contraction of the pharyngeal musculature was essentially nonexistent. There was no wasting or fasciculations of involved musculature. Jaw jerk, palmomental sucking, and biting reflexes were absent. Tests of the tongue musculature proved normal. There was no gross evidence for compromise in strength or function of the trapezii or sternocleidomastoid musculature (supplemental muscles of respiration, cranial nerve XI).

Articulation was characterized by moderately slowed and grossly irregular oral alternate and sequential motion rates. The sequences could not be completed without use of the thumb to approximate the mandible to the maxilla. Articulation in context was characterized by persistent articulatory breakdown secondary to sound distortion and/or substitution errors. Intelligibility was variably impaired. Oral and speech praxis were grossly normal. Continuous moderate severe hypernasality with nasal emission was evident. Incomplete movement of the soft palate as well as posterior pharyngeal wall was delineated further on videofluoroscopic examination. Closure of the nares improved resonation. Voice quality was rated mildly hoarse. Maximum phonation time averaged twenty seconds. Cough and hard glottal attack were sharp. Endoscopic examination suggested normal vocal fold adduction and abduction, although movement was sluggish. Respiratory support for speech was adequate, with speaking rate decreased—possibly to compensate for the articulatory imprecision.

Visual fields were normal on both single and double simultaneous stimulation testing. The patient had no difficulty following the context of examination. There were no language or cognitive signs. He was affectively appropriate and well-oriented to events and surroundings.

Salient symptoms/signs	Test results	Impressions

Worksheet

This worksheet is to be used for recording relevant diagnostic observations. This step should be completed prior to turning to the Impressions. No figure for this case.

Impressions   Flaccid dysarthria involving the oropharyngeal musculature associated with neuropathology of undetermined origin; question of oculopharyngeal dystrophy.

Discussion   The patient's condition had remained stable for a number of years. He continued to refuse muscle biopsy and EMG for confirmation of the clinical signs. In that oculopharyngeal muscular dystrophy is a slowly progressive disorder, this patient's complaint of acute onset of symptoms is rather unusual. Previous neuroimaging studies of the brain, particularly brainstem, have proven normal. The patient has not demonstrated signs of neuronopathy or neuropathy, such as fasciculations or muscular wasting. Moreover, the symptoms and signs have been confined solely to the orofacial musculature.

The oculopharyngeal syndrome, which includes ptosis and dysphagia, usually begins late in life and progresses slowly. As indicated, the cranial nerve musculature is primarily involved, particularly nerves involved in facial expression and deglutition. Both sporadic and familial forms have been reported, with the latter showing a dominant mode of transmission. Electromyographic and muscle biopsy data suggest that the disorder is essentially myopathic in nature and not related to degeneration of associated cranial nerves. Given the absence of fasciculations and overt muscular wasting that typically occurs in neuronopathy or neuropathy (that is cell body or nerve trunk involvement), one could speculate that, in this patient, the pathology is muscular as opposed to neuronal in origin. There is no known effective treatment for oculopharyngeal dystrophy.

A facial splint with a velcro strap to support the mandible during speech and chewing was created for the patient and seemed to help. However, because he found it rather ubiquitous, he chose not to wear it, and therefore continued to use his thumb to facilitate communication and deglutition.

42-Year-Old Female with Adventitious Limb, Head, and Orofacial Movements and Speech Disturbance

History   The spouse of a previously healthy 42-year-old housewife noted that she had recently been forgetting important appointments made only days in advance, had periods of "giddiness," and had become rather impatient with their children and himself.

Previously athletic and well coordinated, she had been dropping things and her handwriting had changed. He had also noticed what were described as "tics" involving lips, cheeks and eyes when his wife was reading the newspaper or watching television.

Although he was unsure of any changes in speech, his children and neighbors had commented to him that her voice had changed and she was slurring words. Discussion of the situation with his wife's brother and sister suggested that their grandmother had experienced similar (and unremitting) changes prior to her death at age 59 years.

Examination   The patient readily interacted with the examiner, although her affect at times was considered inappropriate for the situation. At rest, quick and voluntary jerks involving the perioral musculature, eyes, forehead, and head were apparent. Comparable, although asynchronous, movements were noted for both upper extremities. The movements could not be inhibited upon request nor when resistance was applied by the examiner. Gait was awkward and jerky and seemed to reflect the adventitious movements of the limbs and head. Muscular tone was variably hypo-hypertonic.

Connected speech was marked by irregular, unpredictable, and imprecise articulatory breakdown, with both consonants and vowels being distorted. Some of these errors seemed attributable to the periodic abnormal facial posturing. Oral alternate and sequential motion rates were variably fast-slow.

Speaking rate was comparable to the oral alternate and sequential motion rates, while voice quality was considered harsh, monopitched and monoloud. Oral speech praxis reflected the neuromuscular signs but appeared intact. Definition of proverbs, common nouns, and objects from the same class were considered concrete; the patient was aware of this, although she could not make her responses more complex. Memory for both recent and long-term events was impaired.

Salient symptoms/signs	Test results	Impressions

This worksheet is to be used for recording relevant diagnostic observations. The blank illustration is to be used for identifying and sketching the suspected site of lesion(s). These steps should be completed prior to turning to the Impressions and illustrated site of lesion.

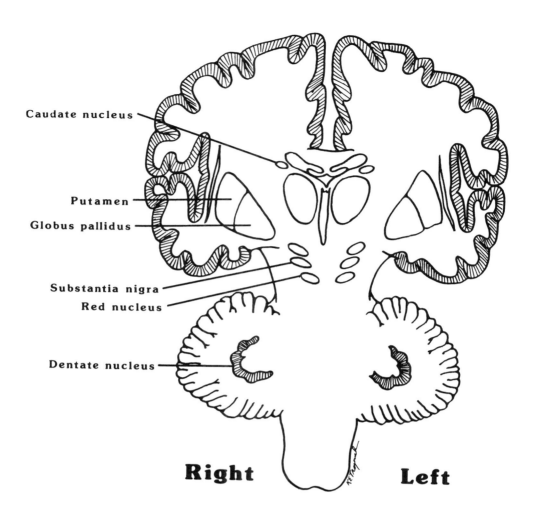

Caudate nucleus

Putamen

Globus pallidus

Substantia nigra

Red nucleus

Dentate nucleus

Right

Left

*42-Year-Old Female with Adventitious Limb, Head, and Orofacial Movements
and Speech Disturbance*

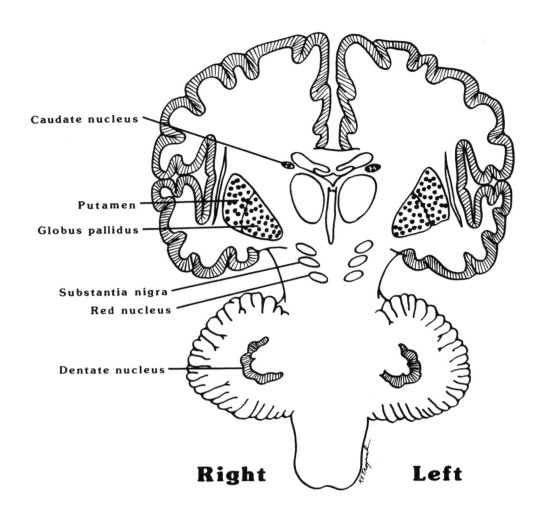

Caudate nucleus

Putamen

Globus pallidus

Substantia nigra

Red nucleus

Dentate nucleus

Right

Left

42-Year-Old Female with Adventitious Limb, Head, and Orofacial Movements and Speech Disturbance

Impressions   Hyperkinetic (quick) dysarthria of Huntington's disease.

Discussion   The matrix of symptoms, signs, and apparent family history led to the diagnosis of this heredofamilial degenerative disease. The clinical presentation of the disorder may vary from one patient to another, with different signs being more apparent at different stages of the illness. The presence or development of marked mental deterioration may necessitate institutional care for the patient.

   Psychotropic agents including haloperidol (Haldol) and fluphenazine enanthate (Prolixin) have been used palliatively for treatment of mental changes as well as the accompanying movement disorder and dysarthria. The disorder typically terminates fatally in 10 to 20 years following diagnosis. At autopsy, cortical atrophy, especially of the forebrain and the basal ganglia, is apparent.

44-Year-Old Male Laryngectomee with Neuropathologic Symptoms

History   A 44-year-old male electronics engineer underwent total laryngectomy and bilateral radical neck dissections for squamous cell carcinoma of the larynx and regional lymph nodes. At the completion of surgery, the margins were considered free. Postsurgical recovery was unremarkable.

On the eleventh postoperative day, a speech-language pathologist visited the patient to initiate postlaryngectomy speech training. The nurses on the patient's service commented that he had been very depressed and was experiencing some difficulty expressing himself through writing, the means by which he had been trying to communicate since surgery.

An intraoral artificial larynx was introduced to provide an immediate means of communication for the patient. Although the patient appeared to understand directions on how to use the artificial larynx, his attempts at speech were marked by effortful groping and intelligibility breakdown. He had a difficult time holding a pen with his preferred right hand. What he was able to write in many ways resembled his speech errors.

Examination   The patient was depressed, but cooperative throughout most test sessions. He was oriented in time and place. Visual fields were full to confrontation. He had a moderate increase in tone in the right upper and lower extremities, with associated hemiparesis, hyperreflexia, and a Babinski sign on the same side. Although he could blink his eyes and wrinkle his forehead without difficulty, the right nasolabial fold was moderately weak and flattened. At rest, the tongue looked normal; during protrusion it significantly deviated to the right and was reduced in strength. Nonspeech oral motor tasks were marked by erroneous placements and groping.

CT scan demonstrated an area of decreased density in the left inferior-posterior frontal lobe region with deep extension into the neighboring precentral gyrus. Blood pressure was 140/110. Auditory, visual, and reading comprehension were unimpaired. Calculations of complex number combinations and writing to dictation were very good, except for the difficulties in penmanship. Spontaneous writing, however, was characterized by numerous misspellings and syntactical errors. Short- and long-term memory were unimpaired.

The patient did not learn to articulate spontaneously using the artificial larynx; nor was he able to imitate individual sounds or monosyllables.

Salient symptoms/signs	Test results	Impressions

This worksheet is to be used for recording relevant diagnostic observations. The blank illustration is to be used for identifying and sketching the suspected site of lesion(s). These steps should be completed prior to turning to the Impressions and illustrated site of lesion.

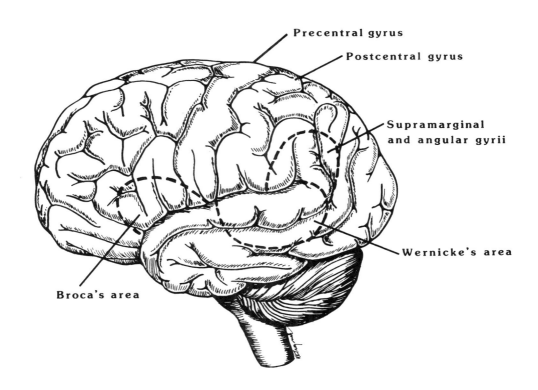

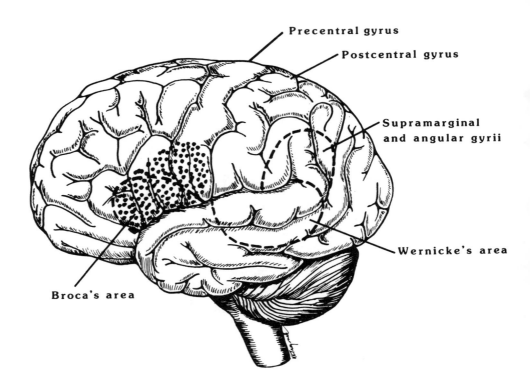

Precentral gyrus

Postcentral gyrus

Supramarginal
and angular gyrii

Wernicke's area

Broca's area

Impressions   Apraxia of speech subsequent to left hemisphere stroke.

Discussion   Our patient was initially treated for laryngeal carcinoma. During, or shortly following, his laryngectomy he apparently suffered a stroke with primary involvement of the left frontal lobe and precentral gyrus.

CT scans substantiated this conclusion by demonstrating an infarct encompassing these regions. A brain infarct is characterized by necrotic tissue, which softens and then liquefies over a period of several days.

A common cause of infarct is interruption of the normal blood supply to an area of the brain by blood clot (hemorrhage) or blockage of an artery. The left internal carotid and middle cerebral arteries are often implicated in those patients whose CVAs result in a speech or language disturbance.

We suspect that the surgical procedures performed in this case were not wholly unrelated to the stroke, and it is likely that an embolus traveled from its origin in the neck region to the frontal lobe.

Our patient's inability to verbalize due to laryngectomy camouflaged his neurologic expressive deficits. Furthermore, because his comprehension was unimpaired, it was not apparent that his difficulty in learning alaryngeal speech may have been caused by more than the laryngectomy procedure itself. His writing deficits and hemiparesis cued us as to the likelihood of confounding factors.

Hemiparesis is usually caused by a contralateral lesion of the pyramidal system. In this case, the site of damage was likely the left precentral gyrus and associated white matter involving the corticospinal (limb signs) and corticobulbar (face and tongue signs) tracts as well as Broca's area resulting in apraxia of speech.

The poor writing skills exhibited by our patient may have been manifestations of both the right hand paresis and difficulty sequencing letters; dysgraphia. We suspect that his failure to articulate even simple sounds using the artificial larynx was probably due to the dyspraxia, exacerbated by tongue and face weakness, and to a lesser extent oral stiffness, as a consequence of surgery. In apraxia of speech it is not uncommon to see co-occuring dysgraphia.

30-Year-Old Female with History of Breast Cancer, and Gait and Speech Disturbance

History Over the course of two years, a 30-year-old woman underwent uni-lateral mastectomy, followed by full course radiation for cancer. Her continued difficulties with gait, and the onset of communicative difficulties, prompted her visit to the clinic for further testing and treatment.

Examination The patient was coherent and cooperative throughout the evaluation. Her use of language was age appropriate, and she gave the impression of being educated beyond her high school training.

Her gait was wide-based and reeling. Alternate pronation and supination rates of both hands were moderately imprecise, slow, and irregular, as was tapping of the right hand and right foot. Hypotonia of the limbs was noted bilaterally, as was a moderate degree of associated weakness of these limbs. Deep tendon reflexes in the right limbs were sluggish. Generalized dyssynergia was evident in which the range, direction, and force of contractions of the limb musculature were improperly gauged (dysmetria) and fell short of or exceeded the intended target (past-pointing). Intention tremor was seen bilaterally on finger-to-nose testing. Upon palpation of the lower back area the patient complained of severe tenderness.

Articulation was moderately imprecise, and varied from periods of slow to very fast rates of production. Oral alternate motion rates also varied from slow to fast, and they were imprecise and especially dysrhythmic. Contextual speech was marred by abnormal and excessive syllable prolongations, intersyllabic pausing, and incorrect accentuation of syllables within various words. These latter features in particular give her speech a slurred quality. In contextual speech, abnormal pitch and loudness variations and mild vocal harshness were noted. Resonance was normal.

Salient symptoms/signs	Test results	Impressions

This worksheet is to be used for recording relevant diagnostic observations. The blank illustration is to be used for identifying and sketching the suspected site of lesion(s). These steps should be completed prior to turning to the Impressions and illustrated site of lesion.

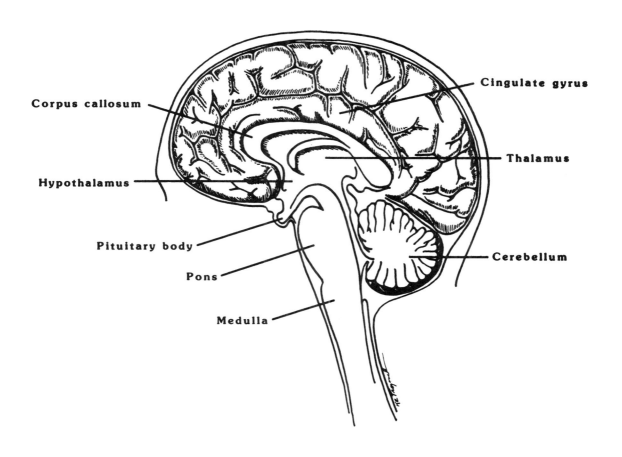

Corpus callosum

Hypothalamus

Pituitary body

Pons

Medulla

Cingulate gyrus

Thalamus

Cerebellum

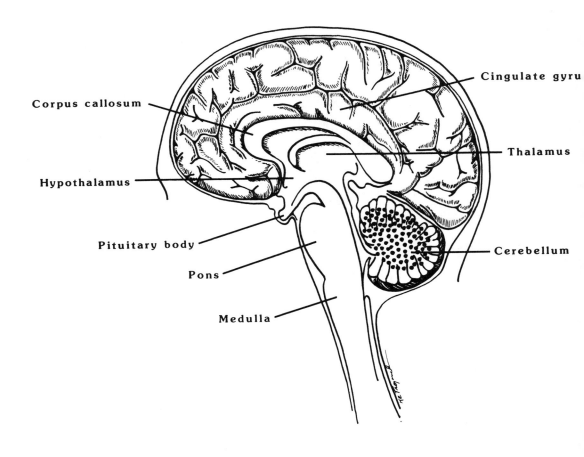

Corpus callosum

Cingulate gyru

Thalamus

Hypothalamus

Pituitary body

Pons

Cerebellum

Medulla

Impressions   Ataxic dysarthria, cerebellar ataxia.

Discussion   The patient's history would suggest metastasis to the cerebellum as the likely etiology for the aberrant movements and speech. The cerebellum: (1) coordinates somatic motor activity; (2) regulates muscle tone; (3) influences and helps maintain equilibrium and body posture; and (4) assists in the speed, force, timing and synergy of muscular contractions that are characteristic of skilled voluntary movement.

The patient's symptoms are typical sequelae of cerebellar dysfunction. The tenderness in her lumbar-sacral region was found to be secondary to metastasis.

54-Year-Old Male with Abnormal Voice After Surgery

History The patient is a 54-year-old male with cerebral vascular disease, who underwent a reportedly uncomplicated left endarterectomy four months previously, and a comparable procedure on the right three days before being seen. Within 24 hours of this operation, he had experienced severe dyspnea, necessitating resuscitation and oxygen therapy, along with tracheotomy. He was referred by the Neurology Service for evaluation of communicative function.

Examination With the exception of phonation, the motor speech examination was normal. There were no language or cognitive symptoms or signs.

The patient was fitted with an unoccluded cuffless tracheostomy tube. Perceptually, his voice was moderately breathy-hoarse and high-pitched. He could produce only a few syllables per breath with finger occlusion of the tracheostomy tube. Laryngeal and videostroboscopic examination (with the tracheostomy occluded) revealed (1) bilateral paralysis of the vocal folds in the paramedian plane, with absence of abduction during easy and deep breathing maneuvers, (2) preservation of the mucosal waveform bilaterally, and (3) incomplete glottic closure. Pitch control could be altered, but phonation time and loudness were limited. The hoarse-breathy quality persisted. Acoustic analysis showed a fundamental frequency of 254 Hz with altered shimmer and jitter, increased harmonic/noise ratio, and decreased maximum phonation time. Aerodynamic assessment revealed increased glottal airflow and decreased intraoral breath pressure during production of vowel-consonant-vowel utterances.

Salient symptoms/signs	Test results	Impressions

This worksheet is to be used for recording relevant diagnostic observations. This step should be completed prior to turning to the Impressions. No figure for this case.

Impressions   Flaccid dysarthria (dysphonia) owing to bilateral recurrent laryngeal nerve trauma.

Discussion   Neurapraxic vagal nerve injuries may occur with endarterectomy because of retraction and stretching of the nerve required for gaining adequate access to the carotid artery. As a result, there may be temporary weakness of the laryngeal musculature on the affected side. The involved vocal fold may show signs of paresis or even paralysis in the paramedian or fully abducted position. The latter position suggests higher involvement of the vagal nerve trunk, implicating the superior laryngeal nerve and its tensing properties via the cricothyroid muscle. It should be noted, however, that acute low vagal nerve trauma—that is, below the branching of the superior laryngeal nerve—may also produce paresis in the abductor position from possible neural shock to the nerve trunk. Therefore, caution must be used in interpreting laryngeal pathology within the first few days of surgery.

Interestingly, in most cases of bilateral recurrent laryngeal nerve paralysis, voice is not significantly altered; breathing is more of a problem. In our patient, this was not true. He exhibited moderately hoarse/breathy dysphonia with a severely high-pitched overlay. We believe that he had adopted a pattern of overcompensation of the cricothyroid muscles in an effort to stimulate improvement in glottic closure during phonation. This pattern may have been promoted further by the presence of the tracheostomy tube and the need for increased subglottic air pressure for voice.

Although we did not examine the patient following the first (left) endarterectomy, we speculated that the left recurrent laryngeal nerve had been affected at that time. The patient did not present with significant postoperative dysphonia, possibly because the contralateral vocal fold was able to compensate for both respiratory and phonatory requirements. It is also possible that any effects of recurrent laryngeal nerve trauma were masked by irritation of the larynx caused by intubation. It was not until after the right endarterectomy with involvement of the right recurrent laryngeal nerve that such compensatory dynamics were sacrificed.

At present, the patient is tolerating the challenged airway and voice. According to the operative note, there was no indication that the recurrent laryngeal nerves had been inadvertently severed. We are hopeful that his disorder does represent a neurapraxic injury, that function will be regained within the next six to twelve months and that he can be safely decannulated.

13-Year-Old Female with Speech Signs and Symptoms

History The patient is a 13-year-9 month-old female who came to the clinic for counselling following the onset of menses. For some time, family and friends felt she was depressed and that her speech was "different." Prior medical history was incomplete in that she was removed from her home because of sexual abuse. However, she had not had any surgeries, been hospitalized, nor experienced allergy to medication. Her only medications included vitamins with iron.

Examination Examination revealed bilateral facial weakness, lips abducted at rest, and ptosis. Lip seal and strength with reinforcement was moderately reduced. Tongue protrusion was symmetrical and to the midline but reduced in strength. Lateralization was symmetrical with moderate reduction in strength. The appearance of the tongue was normal with no evidence of fasciculations. Tongue posturing was peculiar in that the tongue tip was characteristically held against the alveolar ridge.

The soft palate was symmetrical at rest. Upon voicing, minimal movements of the posterior pharyngeal wall, posterior faucial arches, and soft palate were noted. The gag reflex was reduced. The hard palatal vault was considered high.

Lingual and labial diadochokinetic rates were moderately irregular and produced at reduced amplitudes. Variable articulatory imprecision in conversational speech occurred, characterized mostly by sound distortions.

Laryngeal function was marked by continuous breathiness with reduced cough. Indirect rigid fiberoptic laryngoscopy suggested incomplete vocal fold adduction.

Continuous moderate to severe nasal emission and hypernasality were apparent, the perceptual features being modified significantly with anterior occlusion of the nares of the examiner.

Respiratory support for speech was considered mildly weak, while speaking rhythm and rate were variable.

Reflexes were slightly brisk at the knees with absent ankle jerks; toes were downgoing. Muscle strength was normal proximally, with questionable mild weakness of the neck flexors. Hand grips were slow to relax bilaterally. Sensation was intact, and coordination was within normal limits.

Salient symptoms/signs	Test results	Impressions

This worksheet is to be used for recording relevant diagnostic observations. This step should be completed prior to turning to the Impressions. No figure for this case.

Impressions   Flaccid (lower motor neuron) dysarthria secondary to primary myopathy: myotonic dystrophy.

Discussion   Myotonic dystrophy is a systemic hereditary disorder in which myotonia and distal muscular atrophy are accompanied by cataracts, frontal baldness, gonadal atrophy, cardiomyopathy, mental defect, or dementia, hypersomnia, and abnormalities of serum immunoglobulins. The condition usually declares itself between the ages of 20 and 50, but clinical features may be evident in the second decade.

Myotonia is the combined active contraction of a muscle after voluntary effort has ceased. It is best demonstrated as a slowness in relaxation of the grip or persistent dimpling after a sharp blow over a muscle belly.

Electromyography and muscle biopsy are useful in confirming the diagnosis. There is no effective treatment for the disease, but genetic counselling is a very important part of the management.

Myotonia congenita usually begins at birth, but clinical presentation may be delayed for several years. Diffuse hypertrophy of muscles is a usual feature. Myotonia is generalized, aggravated by rest and cold temperatures, and gradually relieved by exercise.

Although it has been suggested that strengthening exercises may exacerbate the muscle weakness and increase the progressive nature of the disease, we have not found this to be evident. Our patient was fitted with a palatal lift prosthesis in order to enhance speech resonation and thereby intelligibility. She receives periodic speech therapy, although its effects have appeared equivocal.

74-Year-Old Hypertensive Male with Variable Language Symptoms

History   The patient is a 74-year-old male originally diagnosed as having temporal arteritis. He was started on prednisone and was doing quite well with regard to the symptom complex associated with temporal arteritis until two weeks prior to admission. At that time, he fell while getting his mail. He denied loss of consciousness, seizure-type activity, or preceding palpitations or chest pains. He indicated that he had "had a small stroke."

He was admitted to the community hospital for observation where he remained for three days. His daughter felt that his speech had changed somewhat during the hospitalization, and that he had trouble finding the right words. At discharge, however, he felt that his communication was normal. Upon returning home, his communication again was judged abnormal, which the family physician interpreted as being secondary to a "mild stroke."

The patient was referred to a larger medical center for comprehensive evaluation. He underwent CT scan, which was normal. He denied motoric or sphincteric problems, but had noted occasional dribbling of urination following a transurethral prostate resection three years prior to admission. He occasionally complained of numbness in the right leg but denied weakness. Futher, he felt that the deficit in speech, which he now acknowledged, and which had been described previously by family members, was not stable.

Besides temporal arteritis and the prostate surgery, prior medical history was significant for hypertension and atherosclerotic coronary vascular disease; both conditions were being managed medically.

Examination   The patient was pleasant and in no distress on examination. The only significant findings were those neurologic in origin.

The patient had a very mild right hemiparesis with mildly brisk reflexes in both the upper and lower extremities on that side. There was a question of a right Babinski sign. He appeared oriented, but variably followed examination instructions and commands. This hindered the neuromuscular examination somewhat. However, gross cerebellar and sensory functions appeared within normal limits. Cranial nerve function was normal. Gait was felt to be compatible with the patient's age.

The admitting CT scan was reevaluated and again judged as normal. The patient was scheduled for EEG and possibly cerebral angiography. Examination of communicative function revealed normal neuromuscular control and motor speech planning; there were no signs of dysarthria nor speech-oral dyspraxia.

Expressive language function was marked by extended periods of normal verbal expression (up to 10 minutes) followed by instances of neologistic distortion, word-finding problems, perseveration, and agrammatical sentence structure. The patient was not generally aware of these errors.

Ninety to 100 percent of the items requiring comprehension of simple-to-complex instructions and right-left orientation were missed. He variably understood the task for assessment of auditory retention, making quantification of these skills equivocal. Of the items requiring recognition and comprehension of pictures, isolated letters, isolated words, and simple-to-complex sentences, 90 percent were missed. Only 2 of 30 common objects to be named were missed, but the patient did not understand the task for assessment of mental and paper-pencil computation or writing to dictation.

Throughout both speech and language assessment, periodic tremor-like movements of the right upper extremity were noted.

Worksheet

Salient symptoms/signs	Test results	Impressions

This worksheet is to be used for recording relevant diagnostic observations. The blank illustration is to be used for identifying and sketching the suspected site of lesion(s). These steps should be completed prior to turning to the Impressions and illustrated site of lesion.

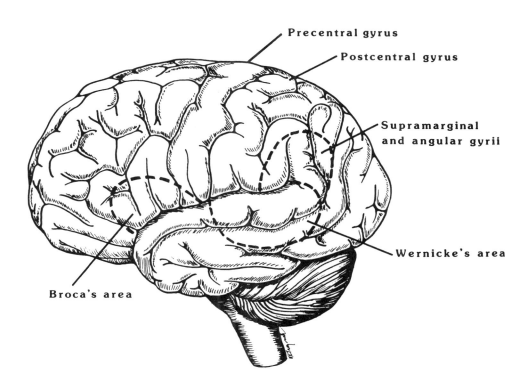

Precentral gyrus

Postcentral gyrus

Supramarginal
and angular gyrii

Wernicke's area

Broca's area

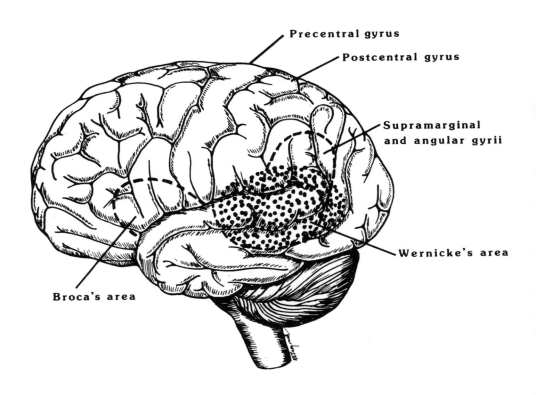

Impressions Dysphasia associated with seizure disorder: Ictal aphasia.

Discussion EEG showed epileptiform activity in the mid and posterior left temporal areas, along with pronounced disorganization over the entire left hemisphere. Repeat CT scan, both with and without contrast, failed to show an associated mass lesion or infarction.

It was presumed that this patient's ictal aphasia was secondary to traumatic head injury after his fall two weeks prior to admission. He was started on phenobarbital and phenytoin sodium (Dilantin), which eliminated the seizure activity and associated aphasic signs.

On three-month follow-up, his EEG was normal. Language assessment revealed only mildly decreased auditory retention, which was considered a factor of his age rather than a sign of aphasia.

Ictal or seizure-induced aphasia should be considered in the differential diagnosis when the patient demonstrates protracted periods of appropriate language function only to be followed by aphasic signs. A seizure disorder may or may not produce motor signs such as arm or face twitching. Finally, ictal aphasia can occur secondary to a variety of neuropathologies including tumor, stroke, and trauma.

78-Year-Old Male with Stroke History and Speech Disturbance

History This 78-year-old male was admitted to the hospital for evaluation following a fall associated with loss of consciousness earlier that day. He denied syncope or presyncope spells, and believed that he fell simply because he was unfamiliar with the surroundings.

Relevant prior medical history was significant for an apparent stroke 20 to 25 years prior to admission, which resulted in a mild left hemiparesis. He had also undergone a transurethral resection of the prostate. Within recent years he had also experienced periods of depression and emotional lability.

Examination At the time of admission to hospital, the patient was taking the drugs chlorothiazide (Diuril) and amitriptyline (Elavil); the latter, according to the family, improved his appetite. Admitting CT scan revealed some dilatation of the anterior portion of the left lateral ventricle, which seemed compatible with an old infarct.

Low density areas in the anterior portion of the left basal ganglia were also noted. Mild axial rigidity was evident. Cogwheeling or tonal changes of the upper limbs were not present. Gait was shuffling and slow with bradykinetic types of movements. A right Babinski was noted.

Examination of the oral peripheral and motor speech mechanism was significant for mildly masked facies and periodic adventitious movements of the perioral musculature. Lip strength with reinforcement was mildly reduced. The soft palate was asymmetrical at rest, being depressed on the right, but velopharyngeal functioning was normal for speech resonance. The gag reflex was also normal. Tongue protrusion was asymmetrical, deviating to the right, with mildly reduced strength on that side in particular. Tongue appearance, however, was normal.

Speaking rate was increased, particularly in short phrases, with short rushes of speech; inappropriate silent intervals were rather evident. Articulatory precision in connected speech was marked by variable breakdowns secondary to sound omissions and distortions, repetitions of sounds and syllables, prolongations of sounds, and periodic instances of phrase and sentence repetitions.

Oral diadochokinetic rates were accelerated and moderately irregular. Intelligibility was variably affected. Laryngeal function was marked by mildly reduced cough and monopitch and monoloudness.

Resonation was considered intermittently hypernasal, while respiratory support for speech was judged to be within normal limits. Language function was considered age appropriate.

The patient was placed on carbidopa-levodopa (Sinemet), 25/100 mg daily, for eight days without significant amelioration of his signs or symptoms. During this period, he was also given concentrated speech therapy directed primarily toward improving the prosodic difficulties, specifically his speaking rate.

Little improvement was noted with therapy. At discharge, the prescription for Sinemet was increased to 25/250 mg, one tablet 3 times a day. He was also scheduled for outpatient speech therapy. Subsequent neurological and speech pathology follow-up did not show significant improvement in any of the presenting signs.

<table>
<tr><td>**Worksheet**</td><td>*Salient symptoms/signs*</td><td>*Test results*</td><td>*Impressions*</td></tr>
<tr><td></td><td></td><td></td><td></td></tr>
</table>

This worksheet is to be used for recording relevant diagnostic observations. The blank illustration is to be used for identifying and sketching the suspected site of lesion(s). These steps should be completed prior to turning to the Impressions and illustrated site of lesion.

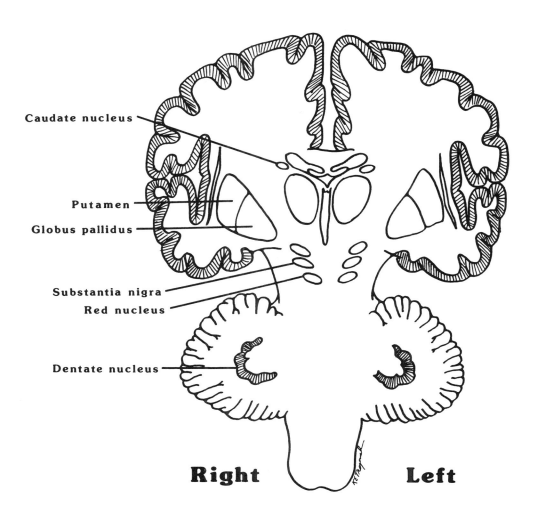

Caudate nucleus

Putamen

Globus pallidus

Substantia nigra

Red nucleus

Dentate nucleus

Right　　**Left**

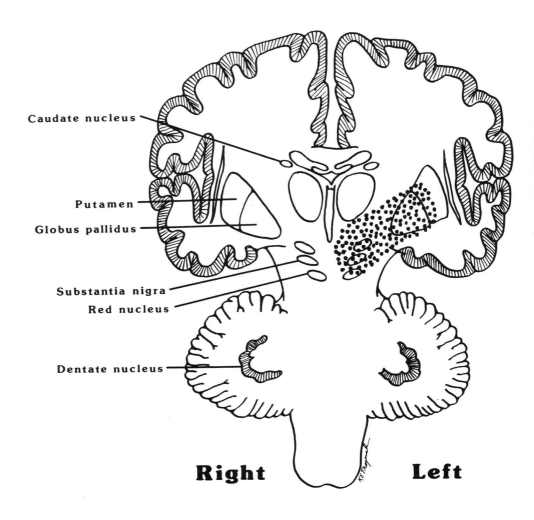

Caudate nucleus

Putamen

Globus pallidus

Substantia nigra

Red nucleus

Dentate nucleus

Right   **Left**

Impressions   Hypokinetic (parkinsonian) dysarthria secondary to a lacunar state.

Discussion   The findings that the patient (1) did not benefit from Sinemet, (2) had a subcortical basal ganglia lesion compatible with infarct, and (3) failed to benefit from speech therapy suggest that his signs and symptoms were due to a fixed or lacunar parkinsonian state, most likely secondary to a destructive striatal lesion.

Unlike idiopathic Parkinson's disease, in which the dopamine-acetylocholine imbalance may be improved with dopaminergic agents, patients with a lucunar type of parkinsonism do not appear to benefit from these medications.

Further, although there is some evidence that speech therapy is efficacious for the dysarthria of idiopathic Parkinson's disease, it did not appear to benefit this patient.

27-Year-Old Female with Progressive Speech Disturbance

History A 27-year-old female school teacher presented with a chief complaint of progressive deterioration in speech associated with what she described as "difficulty making my lips go where I want them to." The symptoms were nonremitting and became worse when she was anxious or during physical stress.

There was no familial history of a movement disorder and she could not associate the onset of the symptoms with any specific situation. She was not depressed nor under any significant psychosocial stress.

Examination With the exception of intermittent, slow-twisting, involuntary hypertonic contractions of the mentalis, quadratus labii-inferior, and platysma on the right side of the face at the outset of voluntary movement, the neuromuscular examination was within normal limits. The posture of these orofacial muscles was virtually normal at rest.

In conversational speech, consonant sounds requiring labial approximation and most vowels were mildly to moderately distorted due specifically to the involuntary contractions and abnormal posturing of the involved musculature. Speaking rate was slowed as the patient tried to compensate for articulatory imprecision. The remainder of the motor speech examination was unremarkable.

Salient symptoms/signs	Test results	Impressions

This worksheet is to be used for recording relevant diagnostic observations. The blank illustration is to be used for identifying and sketching the suspected site of lesion(s). These steps should be completed prior to turning to the Impressions and illustrated site of lesion.

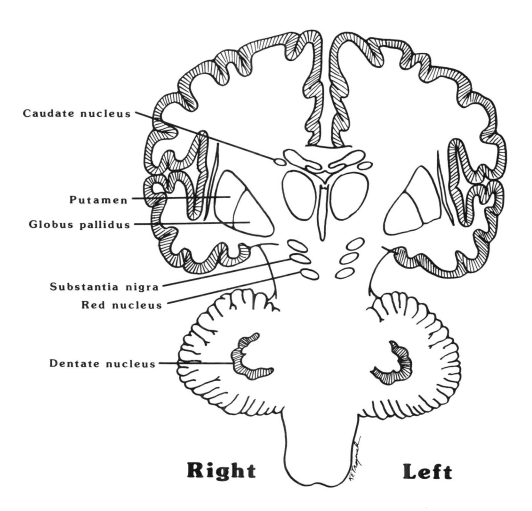

Caudate nucleus

Putamen

Globus pallidus

Substantia nigra

Red nucleus

Dentate nucleus

Right　　　**Left**

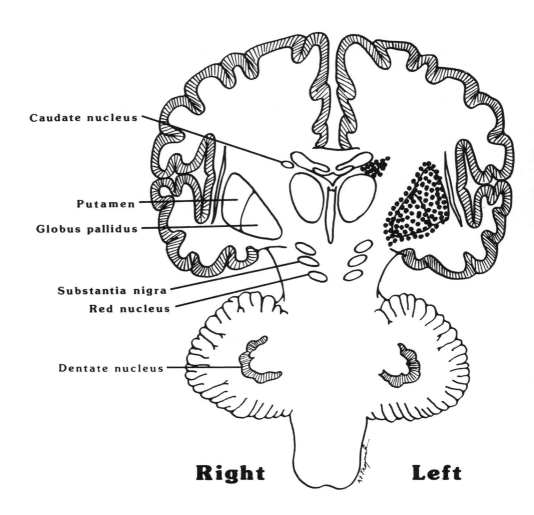

Caudate nucleus

Putamen

Globus pallidus

Substantia nigra

Red nucleus

Dentate nucleus

Right

Left

Impressions   Hyperkinetic (slow) dysarthria: Dystonia (focal mouth).

Discussion   Although dystonia has been associated with lesions of the basal ganglia, quantitative evidence for this is not strong. There have been biochemical studies that suggest that there is an imbalance in the cholinergic and dopaminergic system.

There is some suggestion that focal dystonias, including spasmodic torticollis, writer's cramp, Meiges syndrome, and certain spastic (spasmodic) dysphonias, are early focal signs of a more widespread movement disorder.

Hepatolenticular degeneration (Wilson's disease), anoxia, head trauma, birth injury, and drug intoxication must be considered etiologic factors when dystonic posturing is observed. Our patient's dystonia was focal to the mouth region, the origin of which is unclear (idiopathic).

Botulinum toxin therapy injections are now considered the standard of care for virtually all forms of dystonia. Stereotactic lesions have been deliberately induced bilaterally in the thalamus with variable results. Anticholinergic drugs have been used, with some success reported.

Botulinum toxin was not available to the patient when we first saw her. Speech intervention, however, was begun, with emphasis on lip, jaw, and tongue posturing and articulatory precision.

case 22 — 40-Year-Old Male with Altered Speech and Weakness of the Right Hand

History

The patient is a 40-year-old right-handed male who presented to the emergency room with the complaint of slurred speech and weakness in his right hand beginning four days prior to admission. The patient had been seeing a chiropractor on a biweekly basis for the last few months for symptoms of a chest cold and some soreness in his neck.

Four days prior to this admission, he had undergone neck manipulation and suddenly experienced nausea, one episode of vomiting, and some blurring of vision. Recently he had also noted some clumsiness of his right hand and difficulty walking. His gait, however, improved considerably within 24 hours. He denied difficulty understanding auditory or visual language stimuli, but continued to complain of slurred speech and clumsiness of his right hand.

Examination

The patient's past medical history was unrelated to the present complaint. During examination the patient was alert and oriented. Mental status and language function were felt to be within normal limits. Speech was slurred but intelligible. Cranial nerves were intact. Reflexes and motor strength were within normal limits. Sensory testing proved normal. Finger-to-nose testing revealed past-pointing phenomena with both hands, but more pronounced on the right side. Heel-to-shin testing was similarly discoordinated and more pronounced on the right side. With the eyes shut and the arms extended, the patient had an increased amount of rebound on the right as opposed to the left. Brainstem auditory evoked response testing was normal.

Examination of the oral peripheral and motor speech mechanism revealed normal facial symmetry and strength. The mandible moved to the midline without compromise in strength on elevation and depression. The tongue protruded symmetrically to the midline without weakness. Lateralization was also within normal limits.

A gag reflex was elicited though somewhat reduced; posterior-superior movement of the soft palate was normal, as was vocal resonance. At rest there was a question of rhythmic contractions of the posterior pharyngeal wall at approximately 2 to 4 Hz. On prolongation of a neutral vowel, regular and rhythmic changes in volume at approximately 2 to 4 Hz were evident. At rest, comparable movements of the strap muscles of the neck were also noted.

Indirect laryngoscopy demonstrated rhythmic contractions of the glottic and supraglottic musculature, also at 2 to 4 Hz. Volitional vocal cord abduction and adduction, however, were within normal limits.

Oral diadochokinetic rates were variably irregular. Connected speech was marked by variable sound distortions, omissions, and prolongations of consonants and vowels. Intelligibility was intermittently impaired.

135

Salient symptoms/signs	Test results	Impressions

This worksheet is to be used for recording relevant diagnostic observations. The blank illustration is to be used for identifying and sketching the suspected site of lesion(s). These steps should be completed prior to turning to the Impressions and illustrated site of lesion.

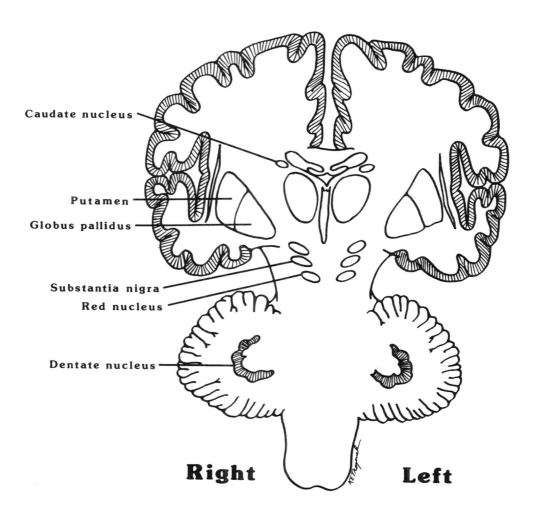

Caudate nucleus

Putamen

Globus pallidus

Substantia nigra

Red nucleus

Dentate nucleus

Right　　　　　**Left**

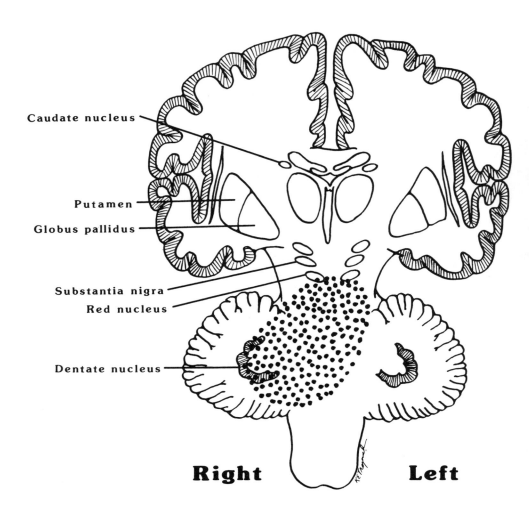

Caudate nucleus

Putamen

Globus pallidus

Substantia nigra
Red nucleus

Dentate nucleus

Right **Left**

Impressions   Mixed ataxic (cerebellar)-hyperkinetic (pharyngeal-laryngeal myoclonus) dysarthria.

Discussion   The patient underwent a CT scan of the head, which showed a bilateral cerebellar infarction, greater on the right than the left. Because of the sequence of events leading up to hospital admission, it was considered that the patient may have experienced cerebellar infarction secondary to chiropractic manipulation. The lesions identified on CT, the clinical signs (particularly the dysmetria in the limbs), decreased balance with eyes shut, and ataxic speech are all signs that substantiate the existence of cerebellar impairment.

The regular movements of the posterior pharyngeal wall and laryngeal musculature, as well as the changes in volume on vowel prolongation, are suggestive of myoclonus. Interestingly, the soft palate did not appear to be involved in our patient, though it frequently is in others with pharyngeal or laryngeal myoclonus.

Palatal-pharyngeal-laryngeal myoclonus (in this case, primarily laryngeal myoclonus) is considered secondary to involvement of the dentato-rubro-olivary tract. The presence of the dentate nucleus within the cerebellum would certainly account for the co-occurrence of these and the ataxic signs in our patient.

Because of the regularity of movement, myoclonus may not be an accurate term for this disorder. Rather it may be a slow tremor. The patient received speech therapy and was discharged on 5 grains of aspirin every day. One-month follow-up suggested notable improvement in the limb and speech ataxia with total amelioration of the myoclonus.

29-Year-Old Female with Progressive Weakness, Ventilator Dependency

History The patient is a 29-year-old, obese, mildly hypertensive female who, on referral from her neurologist, presented for speech pathology evaluation seated in a wheelchair, tracheostomized and ventilator-dependent.

Five years before being seen, she was a business administration major at a local college. She began to experience intermittent generalized muscle fatigue and weakness during normal activity, with her legs, arms, and hands most noticeably affected. Eventually, walking to class and taking notes became quite difficult, and she was often short of breath. At first, she thought that these symptoms were related to her obesity, although dieting proved unsuccessful at limiting them. Over the next two months, she began to experience orofacial weakness, and at that point, sought medical attention. With the exception of a positive tensilon test, the medical examination results proved normal. Her weakness and fatigue progressively worsened in the ensuing months, eventually necessitating a wheelchair and, because of respiratory compromise, tracheotomy and ventilator dependency. Before tracheostomy and because of concern for aspiration, she had undergone a videofluorography study of swallow that revealed delayed oral preparation and transit, reduced laryngeal elevation, and an absent pharyngeal reflex. The small amount of bolus material introduced was aspirated, removed by suction, and the study subsequently discontinued. Because of her course and the findings from the swallowing study, she underwent a percutaneous endoscopic gastrostomy (PEG).

Examination The patient was quadriplegic; she could not move her arms to feed herself. She wore a bib for severe drooling. She was nonverbal. Facial musculature was hypotonic. There was slight limitation of upward gaze bilaterally and weakness of eye closure. Palmomental, sucking, jaw jerk, and biting reflexes were negative. She could maintain an upright head posture.

Evaluation of the oral mechanism revealed moderate degrees of lip, tongue, and jaw musculature weakness and hypotonicity. Attempts at posturing the articulators for various isolated vowel and consonant sounds and combinations showed moderate imprecision but potential for intelligible speech. These efforts were compounded by sialorrhea (increased secretions and drooling). Language and cognitive skills were within normal limits.

Endoscopic examination of the pharynx and larynx illustrated pooling of saliva in the pyriform sinuses, with associated intermittent aspiration. The vocal folds were positioned normally for rest breathing. Laryngeal vibratory dynamics could not be adequately assessed because of the tracheostomy. However, the vocal folds appeared weak and possibly dystrophic bilaterally.

The patient was taking prescribed anticholinergic agents for drooling and medication for pain, gastrointestinal symptoms, and her neurologic condition.

Worksheet

Salient symptoms/signs	Test results	Impressions

This worksheet is to be used for recording relevant diagnostic observations. This step should be completed prior to turning to the Impressions. No figure for this case.

Impressions   Flaccid dysarthria, dysphagia secondary to myoneuropathy; myasthenia gravis.

Discussion   The patient was receiving pyridostigmine bromide (Mestinon) for the myasthenia but benefited little from this agent. Three years ago, she underwent a thymectomy, also a first-line treatment for this disorder. The procedure reduces antibodies in the blood, thus allowing the receptor membranes to recover for transmission of acetylcholine. Response to this surgery is generally good and allows for improvement in the symptoms of this disease. Unfortunately for our patient, the results proved similarly ineffective in improving her symptoms. Since her surgery, she has been hospitalized three times for respiratory distress, as well as both chronic and acute generalized pain. Other pharmacologic agents have been considered in her treatment plan; however, her history of hypertension has limited safe and effective application of potentially useful drugs.

Recently, the patient was fitted with a one-way speaking valve to allow her to speak while on the ventilator; however, she did not tolerate this device. Because she showed promise for intelligible speech, a head-mounted, intra-oral artificial larynx was utilized to maximize her articulatory efforts during therapy. Unfortunately, her prognosis for full recovery is poor.

13-Year-Old Male with Progressive Motor Incoordination of the Limbs, Trunk, and Speech Musculature

History
A 13-year-old male began exhibiting motor coordination difficulties, which were first noticed by his basketball coach. The coach informed the boy's parents that their son was having unusual difficulty with routine ball handling and suggested that a complete physical exam be scheduled. The patient's father had experienced similar motor incoordination at age 20, and now, at age 30, used a walker.

Examination of the patient revealed mild hypotonia and decreased deep tendon reflexes of the lower limbs, and mild to moderate joint position sensory loss. Strength and motor testing of the limb and bulbar musculature yielded equivocal results.

A diagnosis was reserved, and it was recommended that the case be followed carefully over the course of the school year. In this six-month period of time, there was a slight progression of symptoms: Limb activity was clumsier and gait was less steady. Additionally, on exertion he experienced episodes of dyspnea. A reevaluation at the medical center was scheduled three months later.

Examination
The patient was attentive during testing. There were no language signs. Speech production was characterized by irregular diadochokinetic rates with variable amplitude on labial sequences. Vocal quality was mildly harsh; laryngologic examination was normal. Velopharyngeal function and resonation were normal. Contextual speech was marked by variable articulatory breakdown with periodic impaired intelligibility and sound omissions, particularly at the ends of words and sentences. Speaking rate was variable. The variable rate and impaired articulation gave the patient's speech an intoxicated effect.

Gait was mild to moderately wide-based and the lower limbs were moderately hypotonic and weak with associated Babinski signs and generalized muscle wasting; deep reflexes were moderately diminished, as were position sense and two-point discrimination. Heel-to-shin and foot tapping tasks were slow, dysrhythmic, and incoordinated. The distal upper limbs were mildly weak and hypotonic.

Finger-to-nose and alternate motion tasks of the hands were slow, dysrhythmic, and incoordinated; a slight intention tremor was also observed. Position and vibratory senses and two-point discrimination in the upper limbs were within normal limits. A mild degree of scoliosis was detected. Pursuit eye movements were erratic and a mild nystagmus murmur was discovered, but electrooculography results were equivocal.

Salient symptoms/signs	Test results	Impressions

This worksheet is to be used for recording relevant diagnostic observations. The blank illustration is to be used for identifying and sketching the suspected site of lesion(s). These steps should be completed prior to turning to the Impressions and illustrated site of lesion.

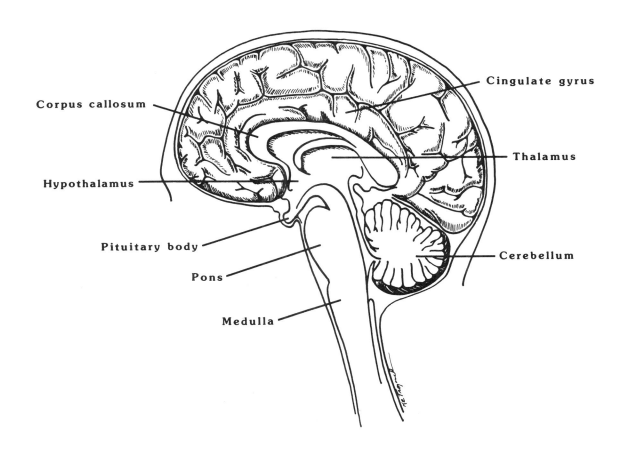

Corpus callosum

Hypothalamus

Pituitary body

Pons

Medulla

Cingulate gyrus

Thalamus

Cerebellum

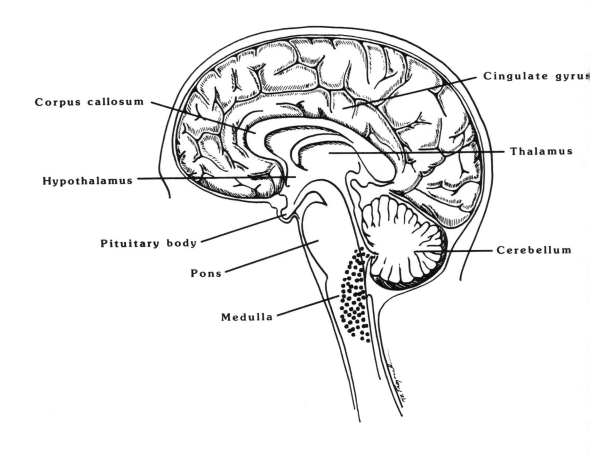

Corpus callosum

Hypothalamus

Pituitary body

Pons

Medulla

Cingulate gyrus

Thalamus

Cerebellum

Impressions Ataxic (cerebellar) dysarthria as a component of early Freidreich's ataxia.

Discussion The term *Freidreich's ataxia* was proposed by Brousse in 1882 and named after a German physician who first reported this distinctive familial clinical syndrome in 1863. The primary clinical features of this condition include (a) onset of symptoms before the end of puberty, (b) autosomal recessive or dominant gene inheritance, (c) gradual progressive and unremitting gait ataxia, (d) diminished or absent joint position and vibratory sensation, (e) diminished or absent deep tendon reflexes in the lower limbs, and (f) generalized clumsiness, wasting, and weakness of limb and trunk musculature. The spinal cord is small due to degeneration of the posterior columns and pyramidal and spinal cerebellar tracts. The dorsal root fibers are also affected and cranial nerves VIII, X, and XII may show nerve cell depletion. Loss of Purkinje cells in the superior vermis of the cerebellum and neurons of the inferior olivary nuclei have been described in some cases and may be responsible in part for gait ataxia, generalized motor incoordination, intention tremor, dysrhythmic alternate motion rates, hypotonia, nystagmus, and ataxic dysarthria.

The dysarthria of Freidreich's ataxia is characterized by: (a) variably slow and imprecise articulation with intermittent prolongations of sounds in words and words in sentences, (b) abnormal fluctuations in pitch and loudness levels, (c) variable vocal harshness, and (d) variable speed and incoordination of lingual and labial alternate motion rates.

Along with the ataxic dysarthria, which is considered a secondary sign, other criteria include Babinski signs, scoliosis, and cardiomyopathy. Although these signs are occasionally evident early in the course of the disease; they are more often present three to five years after onset, and are almost always evident after ten years. Most patients with Freidreich's ataxia lose the ability to walk by the age of 25 years and become chairbound by the age of 40. The mean age of death is reported to be 38 years with a range of 21 to 69 years.

18-Year-Old Male with Closed Head Injury and Language Disturbance

History   This 18-year-old male suffered a severe closed head injury in a motor vehicle accident. At the site of the accident he was in a semicomatose state, and received a Glasgow Coma Scale score of 8. He was rushed to hospital for further evaluation.

Examination   Vital signs were mildly depressed upon arrival to the emergency room, and the patient was unable to follow verbal commands. When he attempted to speak in response to the attending physician's questions, his answers were incoherent but fluent. His eyes remained closed throughout the examination, but opened momentarily when a pinching stimulus was administered. Deep painful stimuli evoked a flexed body posture (decorticate posturing). Bloody fluid was draining from the right ear (hemato-otorrhea) and severe abrasions of the right maxilla were evident.

Sensorimotor testing showed equivocal results. Preliminary cranial nerve assessments proved normal. CT scan revealed a right occipito-parietal hematoma. A right temporoparietal contusion was also suspected. No midline shift was noted, and the ventricles appeared normal with extremely small cisterns. No fractures or mass effects were evident. The patient underwent an emergency ventriculostomy procedure, and was admitted to hospital.

On the fourth postoperative day, CT scan revealed decreased cerebral edema. On the tenth postoperative day, CT scan results were close to normal. At this time, in-depth speech-language evaluations were performed.

It is interesting to note that he was not routinely referred to speech pathology service because the attending staff felt that his speech and language were unaffected. Deep testing proved otherwise. The patient was able to follow simple commands, and appeared to be oriented. Auditory comprehension was mild to moderately depressed, particularly when the complexity and abstractness of the stimuli were increased. Reading comprehension was moderately to severely impaired as a result of a significant memory deficit. Individual written words were easily distinguished, but breakdowns in comprehension were significant at the sentence level.

Visual tracking difficulties, due to a mild left hemianopsia, compounded these reading problems. With minimal cues, however, the patient was able to compensate. Written expression was highlighted by several syntactical, semantic and naming errors. Sequential thought and organizational skills, as well as abstract reasoning, insight, foresight, and judgment abilities were moderately impaired.

Verbal output was fluent, but plagued by distorted and semantically unrelated utterances; confabulations were not uncommon in his speech repertoire. Selective attention and retention deficits were pronounced, and the patient was disoriented, primarily to place and time.

The oral speech mechanism was free of physiological or anatomical abnormalities, and there were no signs of articulation, resonation, or phonation disturbances. Prosody and respiratory support for speech were judged adequate.

This worksheet is to be used for recording relevant diagnostic observations. The blank illustration is to be used for identifying and sketching the suspected site of lesion(s). These steps should be completed prior to turning to the Impressions and illustrated site of lesion.

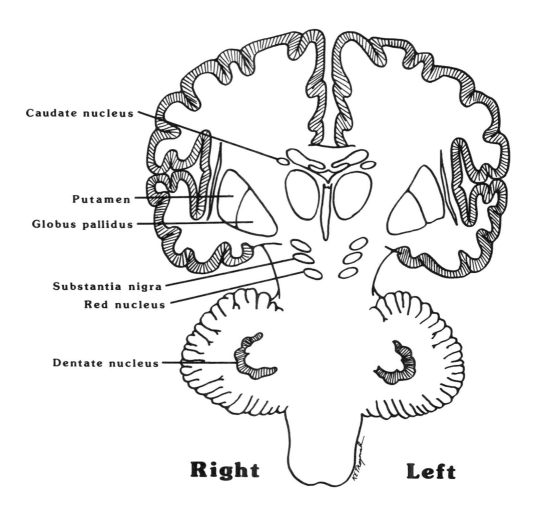

Caudate nucleus

Putamen

Globus pallidus

Substantia nigra

Red nucleus

Dentate nucleus

Right

Left

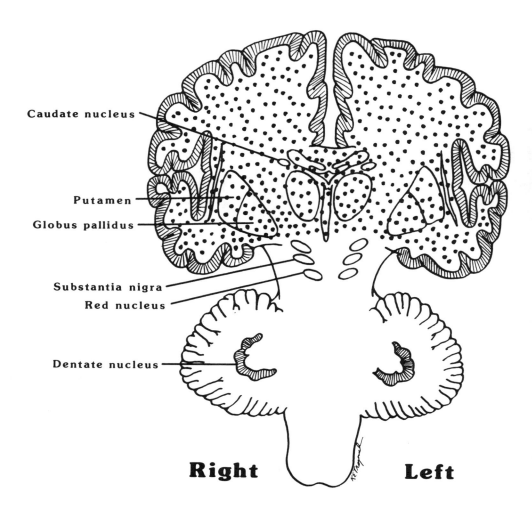

Caudate nucleus

Putamen

Globus pallidus

Substantia nigra

Red nucleus

Dentate nucleus

Right

Left

Impressions   Language of confusion due to closed head injury.

Discussion   Head trauma, whether open or closed in nature, is usually a diffuse process. All areas of brain functioning may undergo pathologic changes, lasting only a brief time or for many years.

Among the most significant of these disabilities include: (1) memory deficits; (2) poor learning skills; (3) short attention span; (4) poor judgment and reasoning powers; (5) spatial disorientation; (6) illogical, confused, and confabulated language use; (7) aphasia; (8) dysarthria; (9) generalized sensorimotor disturbances; and (10) personality changes.

It has been well documented that focal left hemisphere damage may result in aphasia. Diffuse involvement of the brain, however, usually results in disturbances of awareness, memory, attention span, orientation, cognition, perception, personality, and language use, of which aphasia may be a part. These impairments are considered substrates of cognitive disarray and are distinguishable from the complex of symptoms associated with aphasia.

Our patient may appear to be aphasic. His problems with word retrieval, naming, verbal and graphic syntax, and auditory and reading comprehension are not uncommon signs of aphasia. However, his confabulations and linguistically intact statements that are illogical and semantically irrelevant led us to link these deficits to a language impairment plus disturbed memory, orientation, and perception.

The prognosis for recovery of language function in our patient is fair to good. Most patients with similar histories recover basic skills approximately six months postonset. Because trauma patients are most often younger than those who suffer from other types of brain diseases, or illnesses that result in language impairments, approach to their intervention may be different.

Language intervention techniques that can be used with aphasic patients are frequently incorporated into the treatment packages for trauma patients. In addition to these techniques, emphasis in treatment is usually placed on facilitating auditory and visual selective attention skills, memory and new learning potential, problem-solving abilities, and stimulus-relevant responses.

Treatment was initiated with our patient on an outpatient basis. At the time of this report, 10 months postonset, his level of improvement was moderate.

27-Year-Old Head-Injured Female with Limb and Speech Disturbances

History   A 27-year-old female teacher was rushed to the hospital, in a semiconscious state, following a car accident in which she suffered a severe blow to the back of her head. Upon her arrival in the emergency room, she was treated for contusions and lacerations and routinely scheduled for comprehensive neurologic testing the next morning. Additionally, because her voice and speech sounded abnormal to the emergency room physician, a consultation from the speech pathology service was also obtained.

Examination   Although the limb and trunk region appeared anatomically intact, all four limbs were moderately paretic, hypertonic, and hyperreflexive.

The lower two-thirds of each side of the face appeared immobile, with slight associated drooping of the lip corners. There were no other significant alterations in contour or definition of the facial musculature. Nonspeech movements of the circumoral and adjoining facial musculature, as observed in pursing, smiling, lip smacking and laughing, proved imprecise, slow-labored, and reduced in range and strength of contraction.

Although the tongue appeared anatomically normal, it was severely resistive to passive movement. Nonspeech tasks, such as protrusion, elevation, curling, and wiggling, proved bilaterally impaired. Sucking, jawjerk, and palmomental reflexes were brisk.

The velum was anatomically normal. However, during vowel prolongation, velar movements appeared bilaterally insufficient. A moderate hyperactive gag reflex was also observed.

Receptive and expressive language skills were preserved. Consonant and vowel productions during contextual speech and oral diadochokinetic rates were imprecise and slow-labored. The voice sounded strained-strangled in quality, with intermittent periods of phonatory arrest. Resonance was moderately hypernasal and accompanied by episodes of snorting and nasal air emission on stop and continuant consonants.

Salient symptoms/signs	Test results	Impressions

This worksheet is to be used for recording relevant diagnostic observations. The blank illustration is to be used for identifying and sketching the suspected site of lesion(s). These steps should be completed prior to turning to the Impressions and illustrated site of lesion.

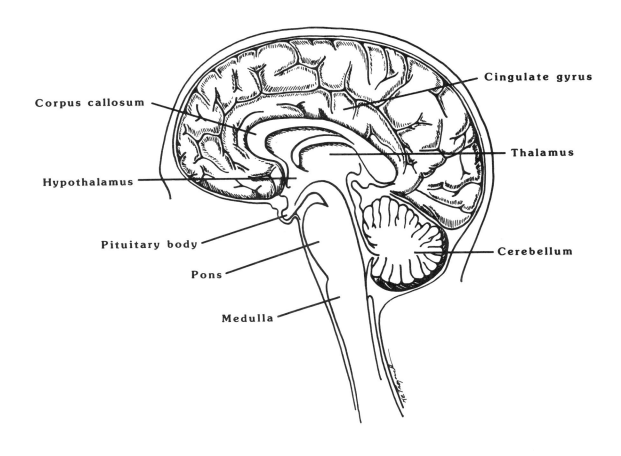

Corpus callosum

Hypothalamus

Pituitary body

Pons

Medulla

Cingulate gyrus

Thalamus

Cerebellum

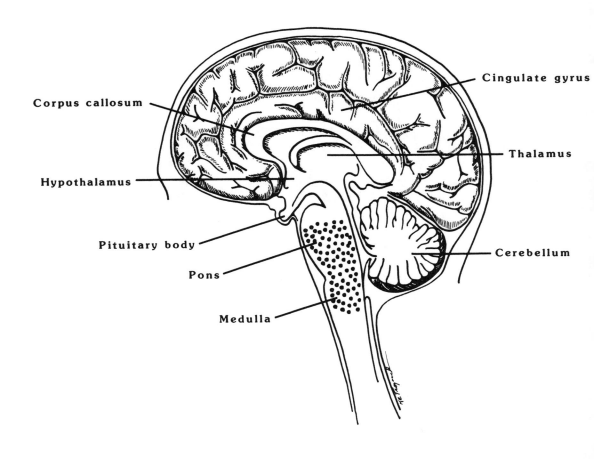

Corpus callosum

Hypothalamus

Pituitary body

Pons

Medulla

Cingulate gyrus

Thalamus

Cerebellum

Impressions   Spastic dysarthria and spastic quadriplegia.

Discussion   The motor deficiencies present in this case exemplify the debilitating effects of traumatic injury to the pontomedullary region of the brainstem with resultant bilateral damage to the corticospinal and corticobulbar tracts (upper motor neurons). The limb and trunk hypertonus and spasticity are principally attributable to corticospinal tract impairment, with resultant disinhibition of muscle groups and reflexes.

The speech signs and symptoms are due to corticobulbar tract involvement with similar neuromuscular phenomena. The absence of abnormal language or praxis signs and symptoms helped to rule out higher cortical levels of involvement.

47-Year-Old Male with Changes in Communicative and Cognitive Function

History   This 47-year-old, right-handed male with a business college degree was found by his mother lying face down but conscious on the floor of his apartment. She had last seen him two days earlier. Subsequently, the patient was admitted to a local hospital where he underwent a complete medical-neurologic evaluation that included CT and MRI scans of the head, both reportedly showing a left cerebral hemispheric lesion. During his hospitalization, the patient experienced mild congestive heart failure that was treated successfully. His prior medical history was significant for protracted tobacco and ethanol abuse that had not been formally treated. At discharge, the patient was taking phenytoin sodium (Dilantin) for seizure precaution (although none had been documented) and a multivitamin. He was ambulating with the aid of a walker.

Examination   The patient was rather thin and cachectic. He laughed or giggled periodically and inappropriately. Cranial nerves V (motor and sensory), VII, and IX through XII were functionally within normal limits. There were no pathologic reflexes. The structural integrity of the speech mechanism was sound for speech production. Articulation, phonation, respiration, resonation, and prosodic features of speech were judged to be within normal limits.

Expressive language was grammatically and semantically sound. He had no difficulty following simple to two-step instructions presented auditorily or visually. Mild dyscalculia was evident; he was not dysgraphic. Visual fields were normal on both single and double simultaneous stimulation testing. He scored above the cut-off on a standard screening test of mental status. Communicative-cognitive testing revealed overall skills at the 88th percentile but significant deficits in the areas of immediate and remote memory. Neuropsychological testing revealed a verbal IQ of 75, a performance IQ of 80, and a full scale IQ of 72. Again, deficits were noted within the areas of memory.

Salient symptoms/signs	Test results	Impressions

This worksheet is to be used for recording relevant diagnostic observations. The blank illustration is to be used for identifying and sketching the suspected site of lesion(s). These steps should be completed prior to turning to the Impressions and illustrated site of lesion.

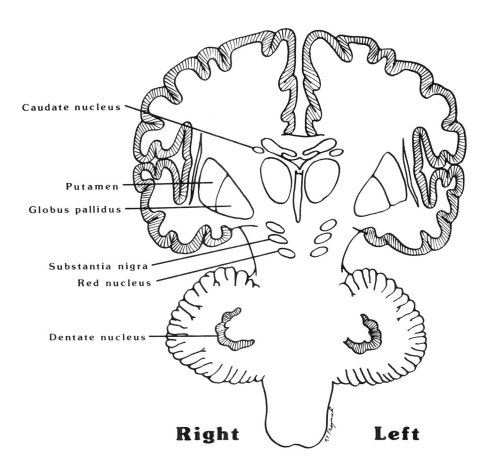

Caudate nucleus

Putamen

Globus pallidus

Substantia nigra

Red nucleus

Dentate nucleus

Right   **Left**

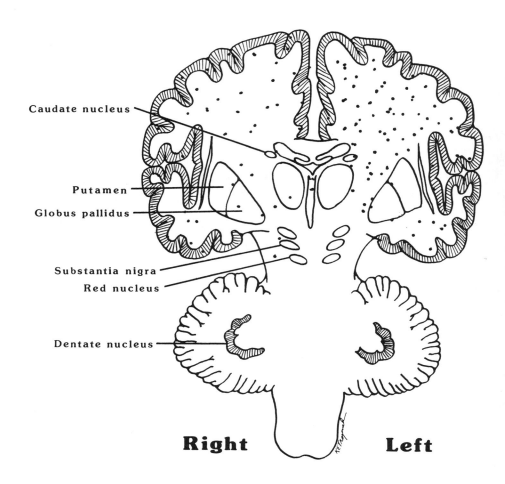

Caudate nucleus

Putamen

Globus pallidus

Substantia nigra

Red nucleus

Dentate nucleus

Right　　　**Left**

Impressions   Mild generalized intellectual impairment (dementia) exacerbated by recent left CVA in a patient with known ethanol abuse.

Discussion   Although neuroimaging studies revealed a left cerebral hemispheric lesion, clinical examination suggested bihemispheric disease or encephalopathy. There were no signs of head or facial trauma when the patient was found. Conceivably, the stroke may have precipitated his fall, which caused coup-contra-coup injury with resultant diffuse axonal injury or shear. One could also speculate that the patient's underlying chronic ethanolism, which can produce an insidious encephalopathy, may also have contributed to his cognitive deficits.

With the assistance of the patient's family members and caregivers, a program incorporating occupational and speech-language therapy was developed to facilitate improvement in both long- and short-term memory. He was also seen by a chemical dependency counselor. At the time of this report, the patient continues to receive communicative/cognitive rehabilitation; re-examination is pending.

62-Year-Old Female with Tremor and Abnormal Voice

History   A healthy 62-year-old female consulted her physician concerning a gradual deterioration in writing, due to what she described as "shaking," and a change in speech, which became worse when she was anxious or fatigued. She was not depressed nor did she complain of psychosocial discord. There was no familial history of a movement or similar disorder.

An anti-Parkinsonian agent (carbidopa-levodopa [Sinemet]) was prescribed but proved to be of little benefit in alleviating the movements of her preferred right hand or the altered speech.

Examination   A postural tremor of the right upper extremity was apparent during volitional acts, including writing, but was absent at rest. Mild rigidity with reinforcement was present in the same limb. Rapid alternate motion rates of both limbs were mildly slow and irregular. In connected speech, articulation was essentially within normal limits, although oral diadochokinetic rates were mildly slow and irregular.

The voice was moderately harsh and monopitched. On vowel prolongation there were regular and rhythmic changes in intensity averaging approximately 6 Hz, which the patient could not inhibit. Examination of the oropharynx during this activity revealed synchronous contractions of the posterior pharyngeal wall, faucial arches, base of tongue, and soft palate. The remainder of the examination proved unremarkable. Thyroid function was normal.

Salient symptoms/signs	Test results	Impressions

This worksheet is to be used for recording relevant diagnostic observations. The blank illustration is to be used for identifying and sketching the suspected site of lesion(s). These steps should be completed prior to turning to the Impressions and illustrated site of lesion.

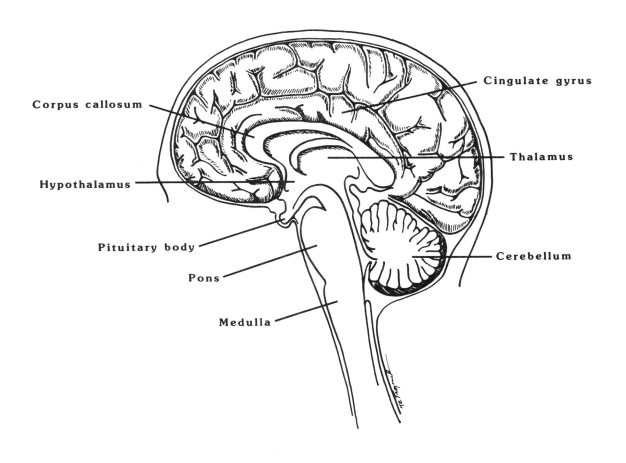

Corpus callosum

Hypothalamus

Pituitary body

Pons

Medulla

Cingulate gyrus

Thalamus

Cerebellum

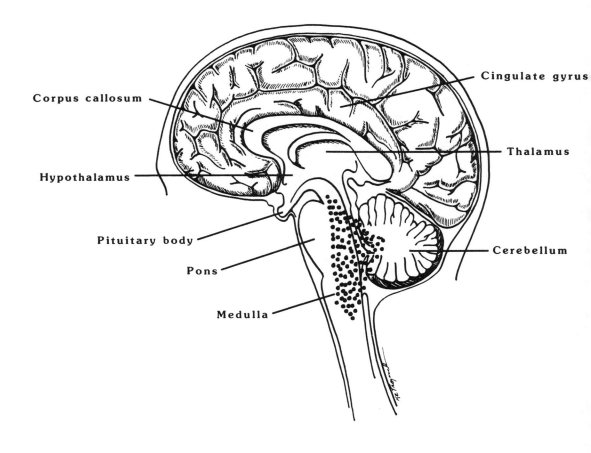

Corpus callosum

Hypothalamus

Pituitary body

Pons

Medulla

Cingulate gyrus

Thalamus

Cerebellum

Impressions   Hyperkinetic dysarthria; essential (voice) tremor.

Discussion   It is not atypical for benign essential tremor initially to manifest itself unilaterally in the arm, hand, or speech mechanism. Indeed, a chief complaint of the deterioration in writing is rather common. Although rigidity is frequently associated with Parkinson's disease and lesions of the substantia nigra and associated tracts, it is seen in the matrix of signs of essential tremor as well.

Although not histologically confirmed, the site of lesion for the essential tremor syndrome—of which tremor of voice may be the primary sign—is postulated to be the extrapyramidal system, possibly within the dentato-rubro-olivary tract network.

Essential tremor may be misdiagnosed as Parkinson's disease or parkinsonism because of co-occuring rigidity and diminution of movement. However, as shown in this case study, essential tremor does not respond to dopaminergic agents such as Sinemet, although rigidity may show some improvement.

The pathogensis of essential tremor varies among patients. It is a progressive movement disorder, more common in males and may be familial. Pharmacologic management has been effective for improving limb tremor. In select patients, methazolamide (Neptazane) may be an effective agent for improving voice tremor as well.

When the speech mechanism is involved (including the larynx), uninhibited voice tremor averaging 4 to 6 Hz, most notable on prolongation of the neutral vowel /a/, with or without voice arrest, may occur in synchrony with movements of the head and the remainder of the oropharyngeal musculature. These characteristics are considered pathognomonic of essential voice tremor.

16-Year-Old Male with Seizure Disorder and Speech Symptoms

History A previously healthy and normally developed 16-year-old male, with a familial history of epilepsy, had two series of seizures: one at age 11, and again at age 12. On each occasion following the events, he exhibited difficulty with speech. EEG studies during each episode showed slowing and spike-wave discharges, most prominent over the frontal lobes.

After the first seizure, low doses of phenytoin sodium (Dilantin) were administered. There were no signs of seizures or abnormal speech within the month period of drug therapy; therefore, it was discontinued. The second series of seizures at age 12 resulted in a long term disability.

Over a period of three years, speech therapy and an increased anticonvulsant drug therapy program were administered. Speaking and EEG patterns were essentially restored to within normal limits. Below are the results of various tests administered immediately following this patient's second series of seizures.

Examination The patient was alert throughout all testing sessions, but somewhat hyperactive. He followed commands, but tended to be easily distracted. EEG was significantly abnormal with bifrontal spike-wave discharge activity. Skull x-rays, cerebrospinal fluid analyses, CT scan, and clinical neurologic findings were normal.

The drugs Dilantin and later ethosuximide (Zarontin) were administered, although the EEG patterns changed minimally. Neuropsychologic testing revealed average nonverbal and verbal intelligence.

Audiologic testing revealed normal hearing and discrimination. Language function was normal. Articulation testing revealed numerous omission, substitution, reversal and transposition errors. Spontaneous speech was moderately to severely unintelligible, slow-labored, and hesitant; there were moments when he sounded as if he were stuttering. Ongoing speech was hesitant with periods of false starts and abnormal pausing and sound prolongations. Voice and resonance characteristics were normal.

Oral mechanism examination illustrated neuromuscular and anatomical integrity for speech production. However, mild to moderate difficulty was observed on volitional oral, nonspeech movements involving the lips, jaw, and tongue. Additionally, sequential and alternate motion rates of these same structures were slow, irregular, and imprecise.

Sound and word transpositions were not infrequent, nor were the episodes of the stuttering like behavior. Complex words—those containing multiple syllables—were particularly difficult to produce. Simpler words were most often articulated with relative ease.

Worksheet

Salient symptoms/signs	Test results	Impressions

This worksheet is to be used for recording relevant diagnostic observations. The blank illustration is to be used for identifying and sketching the suspected site of lesion(s). These steps should be completed prior to turning to the Impressions and illustrated site of lesion.

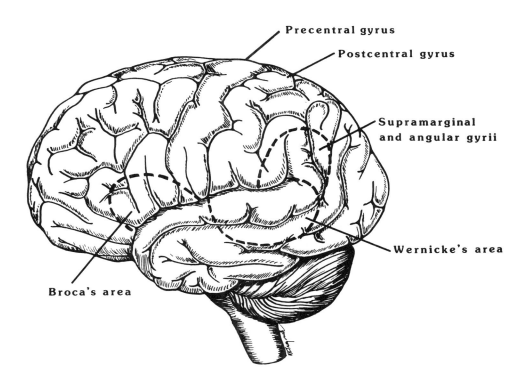

Precentral gyrus

Postcentral gyrus

Supramarginal
and angular gyrii

Wernicke's area

Broca's area

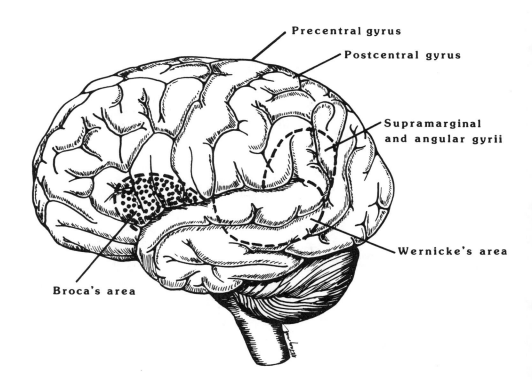

Precentral gyrus

Postcentral gyrus

Supramarginal
and angular gyrii

Wernicke's area

Broca's area

Impressions   Apraxia of speech secondary to heredofamilial seizure disorder.

Discussion   Apraxia of speech is considered by most investigators to be a motor speech (programming) disorder characterized by articulatory and prosodic difficulties. Omissions, substitutions, and reversals are some notable types of articulation errors. Errors are frequently close approximations of the target sound, and they are usually inconsistent and variable. Transpositions of individual sounds, and even whole words within sentences, are not uncommon. Perseverative errors (recurrence of phonemes already articulated) and anticipatory errors (sounds to appear later in the word or sentence are prematurely substituted) are also quite common.

Prosody is slow and effortful and accompanied by audible and visible groping behaviors as the individual struggles to locate the correct articulatory postures for a given sound or sequence of sounds. Inappropriate pausing, prolongations, and repetitions during contextual speech — not unlike that observed in stuttering. However, generally there are no secondary mannerisms.

Apraxia of speech is thought to be caused by damage to Broca's area in the dominant (usually the left) frontal lobe or supplemental motor cortex. It has been suggested that these areas normally function to program the correct articulatory postures for the productions of various sounds and sound sequences.

Our patient's clinical profile suggested apraxia of speech associated with a familial seizure disorder. EEG revealed that his seizures adversely affected frontal lobe brainwave activity.

Three years of speech and anticonvulsant drug therapy resulted in improved speech and decreased seizure activity. Speech therapy focused on establishing gross and fine motor control of the lips, jaw, and tongue musculature, so that he could produce simple, highly contrasted, and easily distinguishable articulatory postures.

Nonspeech and speech sound drills were also utilized. Bite blocks, designed to stabilize the mandible and allow for isolated tongue and lip musculature adjustments, were instrumental in developing ballistic and discrete articulatory movement patterns.

The patient was examined again at age 16, four years after his last episode of convulsions. He was a junior in high school, and had hopes of eventually attending college. His grades were average. There were no episodes of speech difficulty or clinical seizures after age 12, but the patient took anticonvulsants until age 15. The combination of speech and anticonvulsant drug therapy appeared to maximize recovery for our patient.

47-Year-Old Male with Tinnitus, Hearing Loss, and Progressive Gait and Speech Disturbance

History A 47-year-old male construction worker began to hear ringing and roaring sounds in his left ear, which developed insidiously and were intermittent. Three months later he visited his physician because this sensation persisted.

At that time, his physician felt that his symptom may have been job related, due to exposure to loud noise for many hours a day, and suggested that a vacation might give his hearing mechanism a much-needed rest.

Sixteen months later he was admitted to hospital for a complete evaluation because he was having difficulty hearing in his left ear, his gait had become unstable, he had to quit his job, and his speech was beginning to sound nasal.

Examination Physical examination revealed the following: (1) moderately reduced sensation on the entire left side of the face; (2) loss of corneal reflex in the left eye; (3) redness and dryness of the left eye; (4) weakness of the musculature on the entire left side of the face, and associated difficulties with forehead wrinkling, closing the eyelid, and range, control, and speed of lip corner adjustments during speech and nonspeech activities; (5) drooping of the left corner of the mouth, and associated reduction in the definition of the nasolabial groove; (6) weakness of the muscles of mastication on the left side, and associated difficulty in chewing certain food substances; (7) atrophy of the left half of the velum, and associated deviation to the right upon vowel prolongation; (8) reduced gag reflex; (9) mild to moderate hypernasality and nasal emission, especially during production of fricatives and affricates; (10) hoarse vocal quality with associated reductions in pitch and volume variations; (11) unsteady, staggering gait with the feet held far apart; (12) dysrhythmic and variable slow-fast alternate motion rates of the left arm and hand; and (13) coarse nystagmus upon gazing to the left.

Audiologic assessment revealed a mild to moderate left sensorineural hearing loss, with greatest deficits in the higher frequencies; tone decay; and poor speech discrimination skills. Laryngoscopic examination disclosed unilateral left vocal cord paralysis in the open position, and associated atrophy. Plain skull x-rays yielded signs of an enlarged internal acoustic meatus on the left side that was suggestive of a mass.

Salient symptoms/signs	Test results	Impressions

This worksheet is to be used for recording relevant diagnostic observations. The blank illustration is to be used for identifying and sketching the suspected site of lesion(s). These steps should be completed prior to turning to the Impressions and illustrated site of lesion.

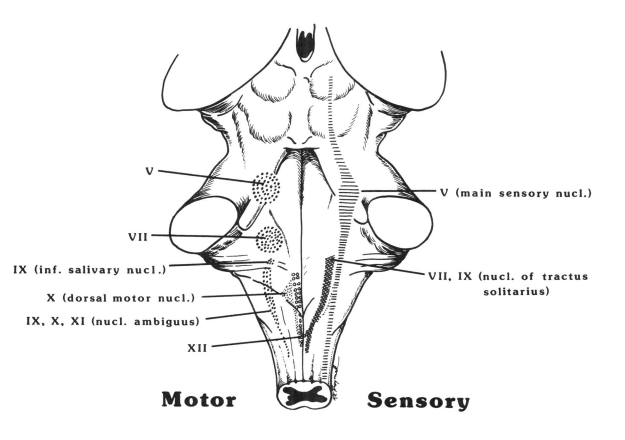

V

V (main sensory nucl.)

VII

IX (inf. salivary nucl.)

X (dorsal motor nucl.)

IX, X, XI (nucl. ambiguus)

XII

VII, IX (nucl. of tractus solitarius)

Motor   **Sensory**

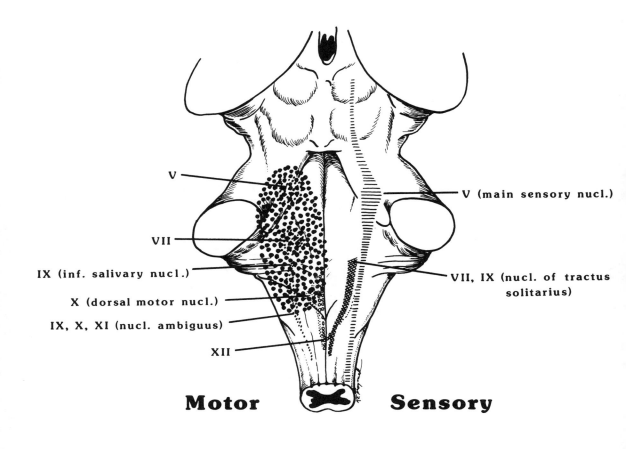

Motor   **Sensory**

V

V (main sensory nucl.)

VII

IX (inf. salivary nucl.)

X (dorsal motor nucl.)

IX, X, XI (nucl. ambiguus)

XII

VII, IX (nucl. of tractus solitarius)

Impressions   Flaccid dysarthria secondary to an acoustic neuroma involving multiple cranial nerves on the left side.

Discussion   An *acoustic neuroma* is a tumor that arises from the neurilemma sheath (Schwann) cells of the Acoustic (VIIIth) cranial nerve. This tumor usually begins its growth on the nerve at or near its entrance into the internal acoustic meatus of the temporal bone.

The early symptoms of an acoustic neuroma are tinnitus (ringing, hissing, roaring sensations) and decreased hearing sensitivity in the ear on the affected side. Such symptoms usually develop insidiously and may be intermittent for many months or even years. It is not until the tumor expands and compresses more of the VIIIth nerve itself, and possibly the adjacent cranial nerves and cerebellar structures, that it significantly debilitates the individual afflicted.

Our patient's early symptoms were classical for acoustic neuroma, but they were not severe enough to yield a clinical diagnosis. As his tumor enlarged it encroached upon many different adjacent structures, thereby interfering with their normal functions.

The Trigeminal (Vth) nerve normally supplies the entire face for general sensory functions, as well as many of the muscles of mastication for motor activity. Involvement of the left Vth nerve in our patient was evidenced by: (1) loss of sensation on the left side of the face, (2) loss of left corneal reflex, and (3) weakness of the jaw musculature and associated chewing difficulty.

The Facial (VIIth) nerve normally supplies the muscles of facial expression for motor activity. Difficulty with eyelid closure and associated dryness and redness of the eye, flattening of the nasolabial groove, and weakness and motor impairment of the lip musculature are all signs of VIIth nerve involvement in our patient. Acoustic (VIIIth) nerve involvement was revealed by the audiologic and skull x-ray data.

The Vagus (Xth) nerve supplies both sensory and motor innervation to the muscles of the velopharyngeal mechanism and larynx. Unilateral involvement of this nerve was evidenced by the atrophy and paralysis of the left velum and vocal cord, and associated dysfunctions.

The velum deviates, or is pulled, to the stronger side during vowel prolongation, and the paralyzed vocal cord vibrates inefficiently during phonation. Hypernasality resulted from velar involvement, and hoarseness was due to vocal cord paralysis and resultant escapes of unphonated air. Compression of the inferior cerebellar peduncle and cerebellum resulted in the ataxic gait and arm characteristics.

Coarse nystagmus is a frequent sequelae to a tumor involving the posterior fossa or cerebellopontine angle. It is unusual that this patient did not also have an ataxic component to his speech. Early diagnosis of acoustic neuroma, as with most other neuroplasms, contribute significantly to successful treatment and cure.

Our patient eventually underwent neurosurgery and removal of the neuroma. Six months following this operation, his symptoms and signs remained relatively unchanged. Had this operation been performed earlier in the history of his condition, perhaps the outcome would have been better.

case 31

80-Year-Old Female with a Three-Day History of a Change in Speech

History This 80-year-old, right-handed female with a history of hypertension under adequate medical control, presented to her family physician with a three-day history of difficulty "getting words out" and "speech hesitancy." He admitted her to the local hospital where her blood pressure was quite labile—210/110 at times and down to 160/170 at other times. His examination also revealed mild right upper extremity weakness without leg involvement. The patient was transferred to a tertiary care facility for further evaluation.

Examination On examination, the patient had no difficulty following verbal instructions and was well-oriented to events and surroundings. Her utterances were limited to "yah" and marginal attempts at repeating simple words. Articulation was characterized by moderately irregular oral alternate and sequential motion rates and significant groping at speech onset. Articulatory precision broke down as an effect of length and complexity; intelligibility was impaired beyond the one-syllable/word level. Twenty percent of the items used to assess oral praxis were performed accurately; limb praxis was unimpaired. Speaking rate was adversely influenced by the articulatory signs and thus variably slowed. Resonation, respiration, and phonation were all judged to be adequate for speech.

Evaluation of expressive language proved difficult, because of the aforementioned findings. She had no difficulty following simple one-step through two-step complex verbal or visual commands (she frequently used hand or head gestures to indicate her response). None of the items requiring a verbal label for common objects or pictures thereof were labeled accurately. In a forced-choice format, however, the patient was able to identify (by gesturing) the correct response and indicate that the "word was there."

Written tasks were omitted because of the paretic right-upper extremity. In a forced-choice format, she had no difficulty with mental computation or spelling.

Mild facial weakness was evident on the right with preservation of the ocular and forehead musculature. Cranial nerves V (motor and sensory), VII (on the left), and IX through XII were clinically within normal limits. The pharyngeal reflex was elicited and was symmetrical. Upper and lower dentures were in place. The structural integrity of the speech mechanism was sound for speech production. Mild hemiparesis and a Babinski sign on the right were evident. A CT scan revealed a low density left frontal lobe lesion.

187

Salient symptoms/signs	Test results	Impressions

This worksheet is to be used for recording relevant diagnostic observations. The blank illustration is to be used for identifying and sketching the suspected site of lesion(s). These steps should be completed prior to turning to the Impressions and illustrated site of lesion.

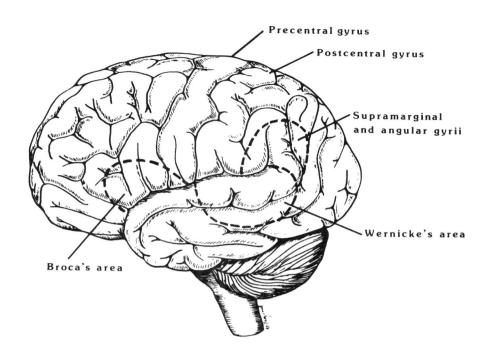

Precentral gyrus

Postcentral gyrus

Supramarginal
and angular gyrii

Wernicke's area

Broca's area

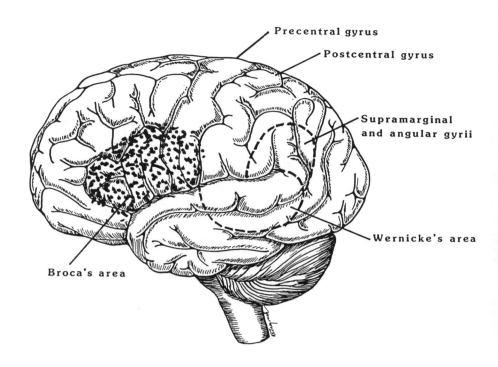

Precentral gyrus

Postcentral gyrus

Supramarginal
and angular gyrii

Wernicke's area

Broca's area

Impressions   Severe dyspraxia of speech/oral dyspraxia complex after left frontal lobe (hypertensive) stroke.

Discussion   The "stuttering" onset of this patient's vascular event is not uncommon in patients with hypertensive disease. As a matter of routine, she had a carotid ultrasound that did not reveal significant stenosis. The patient was continued on antihypertensive medication and one aspirin per day. Deglutitory (swallowing) function, which was assessed formally, did not show significant impairment; the patient was able to tolerate a mechanical soft diet and regular liquids without difficulty. She was transferred to a rehabilitation unit where she received concentrated occupational, physical, and speech therapy for one month. Speech therapy focused on production of simple, visible monosyllabic utterances, progressing to more complex speech as her communication improved. Gains were made in all areas treated, and she was discharged to home with only mild impairment. She was able to express her needs adequately, although intermittent articulatory imprecision proved frustrating for her. She was frequently able to modify or self-correct her responses, however. Speech continued to improve with outpatient therapy.

19-Year-Old Female with Closed Head Injury and Language Disturbance

History

The patient is a 19-year-old female college student. On August 20 she was in an automobile accident in which she experienced severe blows to the right frontal and occipital regions of the head. At the scene of the accident, she was in a semicomatose state. Vital signs were slightly depressed, but stable. No penetrating wounds were detected by the emergency team at the scene.

At the hospital emergency room she was awake but nonresponsive to her surroundings. She exhibited conjugate, random eye movements without signs of papilledema. Rigidity in all four extremities was pronounced, with the legs more severely involved than the arms. Use of noxious stimuli precipitated an intermittent decerebrate state. A full-scale workup was scheduled, and the patient was admitted to hospital.

Examination

Clinical neurologic testing confirmed emergency room findings. Additionally, no signs of cranial nerve involvement were detected. CT scans on August 21 and August 26 showed a marked progression of symptoms of right intracerebral frontal and occipital lobe hemorrhaging. In these few days postadmission to hospital, the patient deteriorated into a comatose state, was placed on a ventilator, and transferred to the head trauma unit.

She remained comatose and ventilator dependent for approximately one month, and gradually became arousable shortly thereafter. EEG study revealed a dysrhythmia grade II, which was maximal in the right frontal zone. Another CT scan showed a right frontal hematoma. The patient developed spiking fevers approximately five weeks postarousal, due to low grade pneumonia.

In late September, the patient began to make attempts at conversation. Spontaneous speech was limited to one- or two-word utterances, most of which were neologisms: she frequently said "stop," "get away," and "don't do it." She could not answer yes/no questions correctly, nor follow simple commands. The patient appeared confused when test stimuli were repeated, or when she was pressed by the clinician. It was felt that these deficits were related to impaired alertness and awareness.

After 98 sessions of speech-language therapy the patient demonstrated consistent ability to follow simple commands. However, complex commands still resulted in nonpurposeful, random, or at best fragmented responses. Maintaining the patient's attention to environmental stimuli remained quite difficult, and required frequent redirection by the clinician. Long-term memory appeared to be better preserved than recently learned material.

The patient was oriented to the year and hospital name, and demonstrated partial recall for the names of staff members and therapy goals and procedures. However, she continued to show confusion about specific test and environmental situations, certain persons, and the order in which activities should occur. Day-to-day carryover was not well preserved. Although her responses were often incorrect due to memory problems, they almost always were socially appropriate or situationally on target.

Matching colors, shapes, and numbers improved, but remained mild to moderately difficult for the patient. Visual motor skills also improved, but remained mildly depressed. The patient could not accurately copy or reproduce linguistic or nonlinguistic stimuli. With assistance, however, she was able to correct her mistakes by comparing her attempts with the targets. Reading and writing skills were still not functional.

Worksheet

Salient symptoms/signs	Test results	Impressions

This worksheet is to be used for recording relevant diagnostic observations. The blank illustration is to be used for identifying and sketching the suspected site of lesion(s). These steps should be completed prior to turning to the Impressions and illustrated site of lesion.

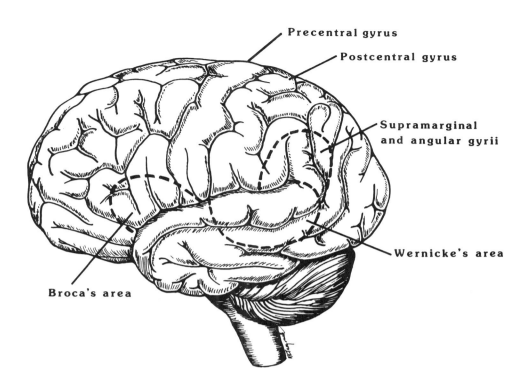

Precentral gyrus

Postcentral gyrus

Supramarginal
and angular gyrii

Wernicke's area

Broca's area

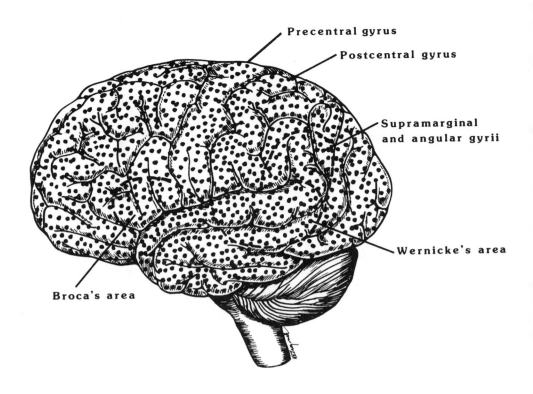

Precentral gyrus

Postcentral gyrus

Supramarginal and angular gyrii

Wernicke's area

Broca's area

Impressions   Language of confusion following closed head injury.

Discussion   More than 7 million head injuries occur annually in the United States. Approximately 5 million head injured individuals are admitted to hospital for treatment. Most are only mildly injured and their stay in hospital usually lasts only a day or so. Some, however, suffer for several weeks from symptoms of impaired functioning, both mentally and socially. Those who are very seriously injured may develop an accident neurosis that can last for months or even years.

Brain damage may be primary; that is, sustained at the time of impact. Later pathologic changes, such as swelling, intracranial hematoma and hemorrhage, hypotension, and pulmonary complications, may result in secondary manifestations of brain damage.

The major effect of brain damage, whether of primary or secondary origin, is widespread neuronal death. These changes may occur within hours after injury, or later in the course of illness. It may be theorized that secondary brain damage is dominant if there were only minimal symptoms soon after the injury, but the patient later lapses into coma. This appears evident for our patient.

Because brain damage is usually widespread following head trauma, neurophysiological deficits are not typically observed in isolation. This is why most head trauma patients exhibit a multitude of dysfunctions of mental activity. It is important to note that whether the head injury is mild or severe, structural changes in the brain may occur, many of which may not be visible radiographically.

Our patient suffered a rather severe closed head injury. Her deficits included memory loss and cognitive dysfunction with associated confused language. Further, there appeared to be a slight personality change in the patient, which became more evident as time passed. Such change is not uncommon in head trauma victims. Indeed, personality disorders and cognitive impairments are among the most disabling of all symptoms. Personality problems also tend to be the least tractable during therapeutic intervention.

Approximately 14 months postonset, the patient could complete structured numerical sequencing, alphabetizing, and sentence organization tasks with only minimal verbal cues and redirection. Moderate difficulty persisted in organizing routine events, regardless of input modality. Routine daily problem-solving tasks remained impaired.

53-Year-Old Male with Left Side Weakness and Speech Disturbance

History   For approximately three months, a mildly hypertensive 53-year-old male truck driver had been experiencing numbness, tingling, and slight weakness of the left side of his body and face and tongue. One day while lifting a heavy carton at work, he collapsed and was rushed to a local hospital.

Upon arrival at the emergency room he complained that he felt dizzy, and that, as in the last few months, the left side of his body, including that of his face and tongue, felt numb and weak. His speech was slurred, but he was not intoxicated. Neurological and speech-language evaluations were scheduled.

Examination   On clinical testing, touch and temperature sensations were markedly impaired on the left side of his body and were slightly diminished on the left side of his face and tongue. Pressure, pain, spatial positioning, and two-point discrimination sensations were only crudely perceived on the left side of his body and face.

Gait was unsteady, with a tendency to fall to the left. Paresis, hypertonicity, and increased deep tendon reflexes of the left upper and lower limbs were noted, as was resistance to passive movement. A left Babinski sign was also observed.

The patient could wrinkle his forehead, but movements of facial muscles on the left side, including those of the lips, were limited in range and slow; drooping of the left corner of the mouth was evident. At rest, the tongue appeared normal, but upon protrusion it deviated to the left. Movements in all directions were mildly limited in range and force and were slow. Other oral musculature appeared unaffected.

Language was considered normal. Articulation was mildly to moderately imprecise and slow-labored, especially during production of multisyllabic words. Labial and lingual alternate and sequential motion rates were mildly imprecise and slow. Resonance and voice characteristics were normal. CT scan revealed a lesion in the region of the right internal capsule.

Salient symptoms/signs	Test results	Impressions

This worksheet is to be used for recording relevant diagnostic observations. The blank illustration is to be used for identifying and sketching the suspected site of lesion(s). These steps should be completed prior to turning to the Impressions and illustrated site of lesion.

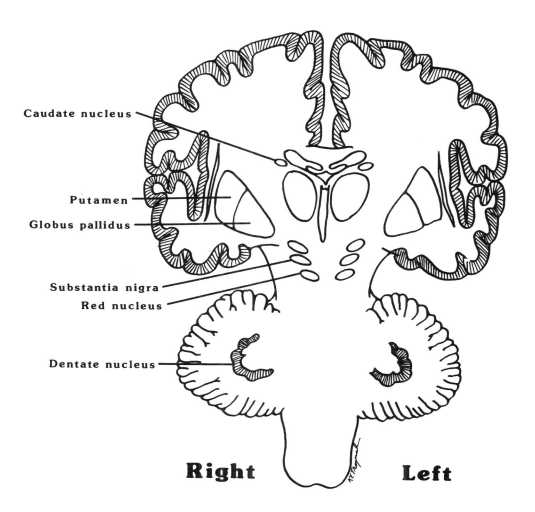

Caudate nucleus

Putamen

Globus pallidus

Substantia nigra

Red nucleus

Dentate nucleus

Right

Left

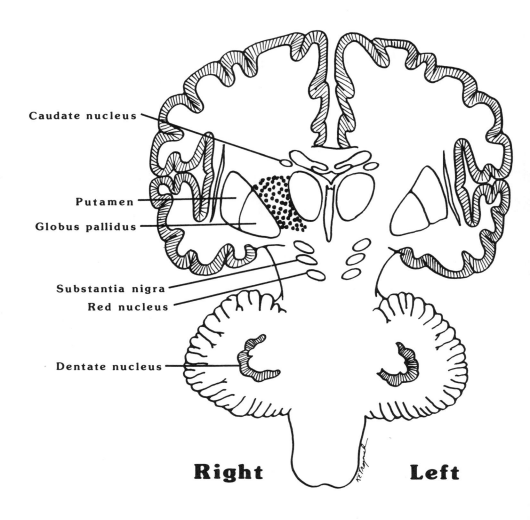

Caudate nucleus

Putamen

Globus pallidus

Substantia nigra
Red nucleus

Dentate nucleus

Right　　　　　　**Left**

Impressions Unilateral upper motor neuron dysarthria and left hemiparesis.

Discussion This patient suffered a hemorrhagic infarct of the internal capsule caused by occlusion of the thalamostriate branches of the right middle cerebral artery. The sensory disturbances observed suggest that damage occurred in the posterior limb of the right internal capsule through which spinocortical and spinothalamic fibers ascend. The spastic hemiparesis of the left arm and leg also implicate the posterior limb of the capsule through which corticospinal fibers descend; and the motor speech difficulties observed are due to damage to the genu through which corticobulbar fibers descend.

A unilateral lesion of the corticospinal tract, above its level of decussation in the medulla, causes contralateral spastic hemiplegia, as in this case. However, the neuromuscular effects of a unilateral corticobulbar tract lesion are not always as predictable.

There is evidence that suggests that both the facial and hypoglossal nuclei receive the majority of their supranuclear innervation from contralateral corticobulbar tract fibers. Consequently, muscles of the face and tongue, which are respectively supplied by the Facial and Hypoglossal nerves, are susceptible to paresis following unilateral corticobulbar tract damage, as in this case. The musculature, however, is not truly spastic in the neuromuscular sense. Labial and lingual movements during articulation and alternate motion rates may be variably incoordinated, imprecise, and slow. Sometimes speech sounds "slurred" or ataxiclike, owing perhaps to the incoordination effects of unilateral muscular involvement.

44-Year-Old Female with Intermittent Headache, Blurred Vision, and Gait and Speech Disturbances

History   The patient is a 44-year-old right-handed female who has a rather vast neurologic history dating back approximately 15 years prior to present admission. At that time she had a rather dramatic onset of symptoms including dizziness, blurring of vision, and change in speech. She also had difficulty with balance and clumsiness, particularly of the lower extremities.

On this admission, her primary complaints included intermittent headaches, blurring of vision, and change in speech. Also problematic were the symptoms of numbness of the left face and tongue; decreasing hearing, confirmed audiometrically, in the left ear for the last seven years; numbness of the entire body especially on the left side; stiffness, weakness, clumsiness; and poor balance in both lower extremities, but greater on the left than the right.

Examination   The patient had bilateral optic atrophy, left greater than the right, with loss of the retinal nerve fiber layer. She demonstrated decreased sensation over the left half of the face. The jawjerk was brisk. Cranial nerves were intact. Muscular examination revealed spasticity of all four extremities, more pronounced on the left side. Both gross and fine finger movements were poor bilaterally. Marked weakness of the left lower extremity was evident, as was decreased sensation in the left half of body. Bilateral hyperreflexia, left greater than right, and bilateral Babinski signs were detected. She has a spastic wide gait and poor balance control.

CT scan revealed multiple white matter lesions in the periventricular region.

The lips were symmetrical at rest without compromise in abduction or adduction with reinforcement. The tongue protruded to the midline without compromise in precision of movement or strength. The soft palate was symmetrical at rest and during phonation. The gag reflex, however, was considered brisk.

Oral diadochokinetic rates were irregular and slow. Articulatory precision in connected speech was marked by variable breakdown, with impaired intelligibility due primarily to sound distortion. Cough and hard glottal attack were sharp. Voice quality in contextual speech and on vowel prolongation was considered strain-strangled. There was a question of occasional mild hypernasality with nasal emission. Respiration was considered adequate for speech, while speaking rate was considered variably fast-slow.

Salient symptoms/signs	Test results	Impressions

This worksheet is to be used for recording relevant diagnostic observations. The blank illustration is to be used for identifying and sketching the suspected site of lesion(s). These steps should be completed prior to turning to the Impressions and illustrated site of lesion.

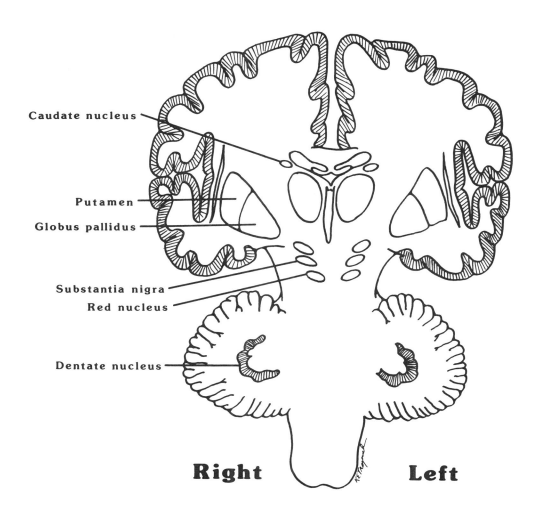

Caudate nucleus

Putamen

Globus pallidus

Substantia nigra

Red nucleus

Dentate nucleus

Right   **Left**

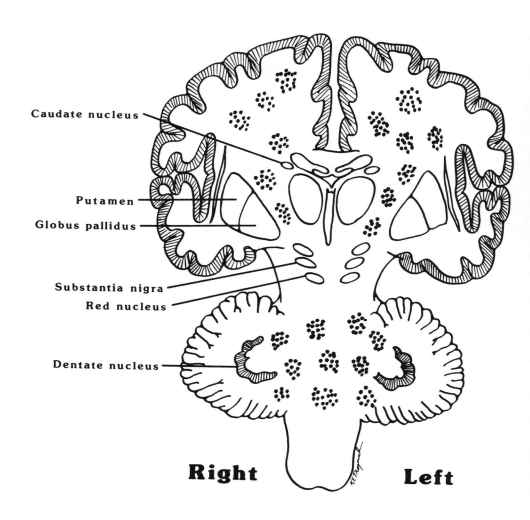

Caudate nucleus

Putamen

Globus pallidus

Substantia nigra

Red nucleus

Dentate nucleus

Right　　　　　　　**Left**

Impressions   Mixed dysarthria of the ataxic (cerebellar)-spastic (bilateral upper motor neuron) types.

Discussion   The history, and the neurologic and speech pathology findings were characteristic of demyelinating disease—that is, multiple sclerosis with mixed dysarthria.

Involvement of the corticospinal tracts (supranuclear) produces characteristic spasticity and weakness. Our patient's spasticity in all extremities suggested such a pathology. Decreased sensation, particularly on the left, involving both the axial and appendicular skeleton was due to involvement of sensory tracts.

Coarse intention tremor and incoordination of the extremities, irregular oral diadochokinetic rates, and variable speaking rate are typical sequelae of cerebellar lesions.

Multiple sclerosis (MS) is characterized by remissions and exacerbations of symptoms and signs. Initially, the manifestations may be subtle and remit quickly, while as time progresses they may become more widespread and longstanding. Clinically, the presence of exacerbations and remissions helps determine the diagnosis.

Although MS is considered a white matter disease, frequently the sclerotic plaques encroach upon cortical gray matter, but do not destroy nerve cells. Histologically, the myelin sheath of axons undergoes destruction (demyelinization) to varying degrees.

The etiology of MS is unknown. Current research suggests that environmental and immunological mechanisms may be involved. While there is no effective treatment available for the disease itself, many of the symptoms and neurological deficits can be treated individually, and the quality of life improved.

58-Year-Old Female with Known Cerebral Vascular Disease, Change in Communicative and Cognitive Function

History

This 58-year-old, right-handed, housewife with a history of hypertension and cerebral vascular disease with right CVA and consequent seizure disorder underwent a right-side endarterectomy three months after a right cerebral hemispheric stroke. Three days after discharge from the hospital, she was discovered on the bathroom floor having a generalized tonic/clonic seizure. She was admitted to the emergency room of a local hospital where she was started on I.V. valium (Diazepam) that stopped the seizures. An MRI scan of the head was obtained, the results of which were pending at the time of speech-language evaluation. Carotid ultrasound was inconclusive secondary to edema; cerebral angiography did not reveal occlusion or evidence of thrombus. Repeat EEG was positive for a seizure disorder. She was subsequently started on phenytoin sodium (Dilantin) to control seizure activity.

Examination

The patient was alert, communicative, and well-oriented to events and surroundings. She commented that her memory was "shot."

Mild weakness of the lower 2/3 of the face on the left, bilateral positive palmomental, jaw jerk, and sucking reflexes were evident. Upper and lower dentures were in place. Oral alternate and sequential motion rates were mildly irregular; otherwise articulation, phonation, respiration, resonation, and prosody findings were not impressive.

Expressive language was characterized by increased response time and difficulty with concept generalization and abstraction. Utterances were grammatically and generally semantically sound.

Of the items requiring comprehension of one-step through two-step complex commands, 100 percent were accurate, while comprehension and retention of a multiple word complex paragraph showed 80 percent accuracy. A left visual field defect was evident on both single and double simultaneous stimulation testing. None of the items requiring visual comprehension or retention of isolated letters through simple to complex words and sentences were missed. Visual comprehension and retention of a multiple-word, complex paragraph showed 75 percent accuracy. None of the items used on a confrontation naming task were missed. Mild dyscalculia and dysgraphia were evident.

Performance on communicative-cognitive measures averaged at the 85th percentile, with neuropsychological testing revealing a performance IQ of 75 and a verbal IQ of 84. On the former, the patient showed significant deficits in the areas of visual spatial skills, visual sequencing, and spatial integration. Moreover, she was consistently below the 20th percentile on measures of verbal and visual memory.

Salient symptoms/signs	Test results	Impressions

This worksheet is to be used for recording relevant diagnostic observations. The blank illustration is to be used for identifying and sketching the suspected site of lesion(s). These steps should be completed prior to turning to the Impressions and illustrated site of lesion.

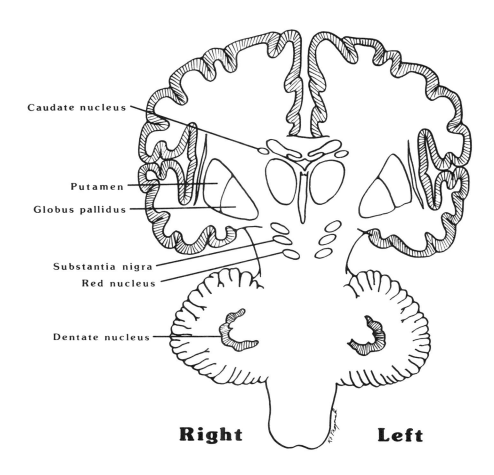

Caudate nucleus

Putamen

Globus pallidus

Substantia nigra
Red nucleus

Dentate nucleus

Right   **Left**

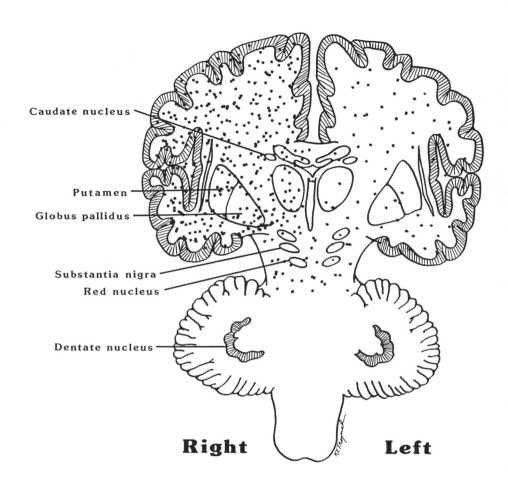

Caudate nucleus

Putamen

Globus pallidus

Substantia nigra

Red nucleus

Dentate nucleus

Right   **Left**

Impressions Generalized intellectual impairment in a patient with known cerebral vascular disease, status post-right CVA. Multi-infarct dementia, moderate in degree.

Discussion The MRI of the head revealed, along with the old right CVA, multiple lacunes (small strokes) within the brainstem, cerebral white matter, and basal ganglia. The ventricles were enlarged suggesting generalized cerebral atrophy. The EEG showed diffuse bihemispheric slowing consistent with encephalopathy.

It is conceivable that the patient experienced an embolic event shortly after the carotid endarterectomy. This may have resulted in an exacerbation of the right cerebral hemispheric signs, such as spatial-perceptual deficits, left visual field defect, as well as generalized diminished cognitive function. During her hospitalization, she received communicative/cognitive, occupational, and physical therapy. Repeat speech-language and neuropsychological evaluations before discharge revealed little change in her neurocognitive status. Her seizures were being adequately controlled with Dilantin, phenobarbital, and carbamazepine (Tegretol). Repeat examination at six months showed slight improvement in her neurocommunicative-cognitive status, although not enough to warrant continued formal therapy. She has remained seizure-free on anticonvulsant medication and continues to be followed by her internist.

69-Year-Old Female with Progressive Speech and Swallowing Disturbances

History A 69-year-old widow complained of dull, aching cramps in her hands and feet, and progressive, rapid deterioration of her speech and swallowing abilities over the course of three months. By the time she was examined, two weeks later, she was also experiencing intermittent nasal regurgitation of liquids, increased cramping sensations in the legs, and more noticeable speech difficulties.

Examination In March, the patient underwent medical and speech diagnostic testing.
Clinical findings included: (1) mild to moderate bilateral weakness of all four limbs, with associated mild hyperreflexes and atrophy; (2) strong sucking reflex; (3) bilateral paresis of the facial and velopharyngeal musculature, with associated limitations in the range, speed, and control of lip and palate activities; (4) hyperactive gag reflex; (5) nasal regurgitation of liquids; (6) drooling; (7) bilateral atrophy, fasciculations, and weakness of the tongue musculature; (8) severely slow and imprecise articulation; (9) hypernasality and nasal snorting; (10) strained-strangled phonation and wet hoarseness; and (11) severely reduced lingual and labial alternate motion rates.

Salient symptoms/signs	Test results	Impressions

This worksheet is to be used for recording relevant diagnostic observations. The blank illustration is to be used for identifying and sketching the suspected site of lesion(s). These steps should be completed prior to turning to the Impressions and illustrated site of lesion.

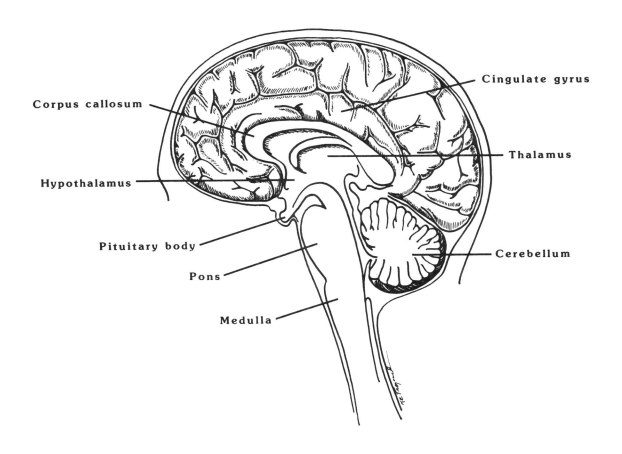

Corpus callosum

Cingulate gyrus

Hypothalamus

Thalamus

Pituitary body

Pons

Cerebellum

Medulla

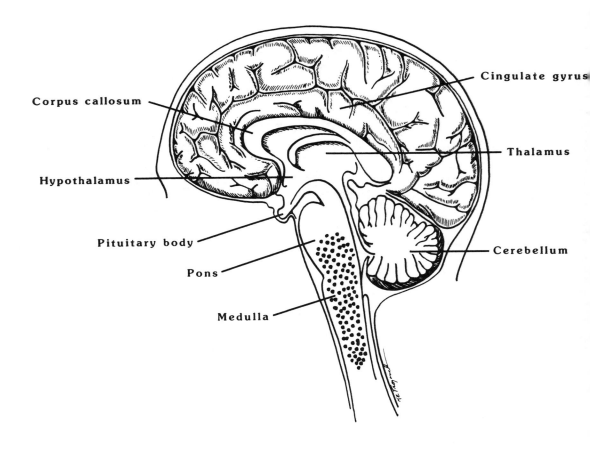

Corpus callosum

Cingulate gyrus

Thalamus

Hypothalamus

Pituitary body

Pons

Medulla

Cerebellum

Impressions   Mixed spastic-flaccid dysarthria due to progressive motor neuron disease.

Discussion   Amyotrophic lateral sclerosis is a degenerative disease of the motor system. The pathology involves the corticospinal tracts as well as the motor neurons in the brain stem and spinal cord. If the lateral columns in the spinal cord are predominantly affected, the condition is referred to as primary lateral sclerosis, and patients present with spasticity and weakness. On the other hand, if the primary site of involvement is the anterior horn of the spinal cord, muscle wasting, weakness, and flaccidity are found and the diagnosis of progressive spinal muscular atrophy is made. Some patients present with speech and swallowing difficulties due to early involvement of the brainstem motor nuclei and are said to have progressive bulbar palsy. In practice, then, three forms seldom occur in isolation; the vast majority of patients having a mixture of upper and lower motor neuron findings as well as progressive bulbar palsy. Most cases occur sporadically, but a familial form of the disorder is also well documented in the literature. The etiology is unknown and there is no cure at this time. Supportive measures to improve the quality of life are becoming available, e.g., portable respirators and augmentative communication systems.

Six months after initial examination, the patient exhibited severe weakness and paralysis of the limbs, trunk, and speech musculature. Such disturbances were accompanied by hypoactive reflexes and atrophic changes of many of these structures, owing to substantial progression of lower motor neuron involvement. Speech was markedly unintelligible due to severe articulatory imprecision, hypernasality, nasal snorting, and strained-strangled phonation.

The rate of progression in this case was rapid. We recommended that nasogastric feeding be used to facilitate food intake, since oral manipulation of foods was difficult. Additionally, she was placed on a respirator, and an augmentative communication system introduced.

45-Year-Old Female with Acute Onset of Right Limb Weakness and Speech Disturbance

History

The patient is a 45-year-old female factory worker who was admitted to the emergency room following an acute onset of right facial droop, right arm weakness and an inability to speak four hours prior to admission. The patient did not have a history of hypertension, head-ache, or previous strokes. Her husband reported that she has complained of a transient "funny feeling" in the right arm during the preceding summer.

There was a strong family history of cardiovascular disease. With the exception of drinking an occasional glass of beer, smoking one and one-half to two packages of cigarettes per day for 20 years, and long-standing sinus problems, the patient's prior medical history was negative.

Examination

The patient was a well-developed, somewhat obese female in no acute distress. She responded well to all instructions. Eyes, ears, nose, and throat were normal. Fundoscopic examination revealed normal discs and vessels. Visual fields were intact with no evidence of hemianopsia. Periodic mucus nasal drainage was noted. Dentition was in good repair. Carotids were normal without bruits. Cardiac examination was without murmur or gallop. There was marked right central facial and lingual paresis. Cranial nerve examination was within normal limits.

She did complain of some difficulty swallowing, although the gag reflex, pharyngeal sensation, and indirect mirror laryngoscopy were normal. She had definite right arm and leg weakness with brisk deep tendon reflexes and Babinski sign on that side. Right pronator drift was evident with eyes closed. Cerebellar function appeared normal. There were no objective sensory findings.

Sixty percent of the items used to assess oral praxis were missed. Oral diadochokinetic and sequential motion rates were slow and grossly irregular, particularly for those sounds requiring consecutive lingual activity. Attempts at repetition of isolated vowels and monosyllabic words were marked by variable distortion, substitution, transposition of speech sounds, as well as voiced-voiceless transposition on cognate pairs such as **p/b**. Articulatory groping as well as variable breakdowns were apparent.

Conversational speech was grossly unintelligible. Speaking rate was characterized by prolongations of intersyllabic/interword intervals, in-appropriate silent intervals, and short phrases. Voice initiation was difficult; however, once produced, periodic instances of hypernasality were noted. Speech breathing mechanics appeared adequate. Dynamic videofluorographic study of swallow revealed discoordinated movements at the oral stage. Clinically, masticatory and deglutitory movements were awkward and, at times, unrelated to the swallowing act. Both CT scan and EEG were normal .

Salient symptoms/signs	Test results	Impressions

This worksheet is to be used for recording relevant diagnostic observations. The blank illustration is to be used for identifying and sketching the suspected site of lesion(s). These steps should be completed prior to turning to the Impressions and illustrated site of lesion.

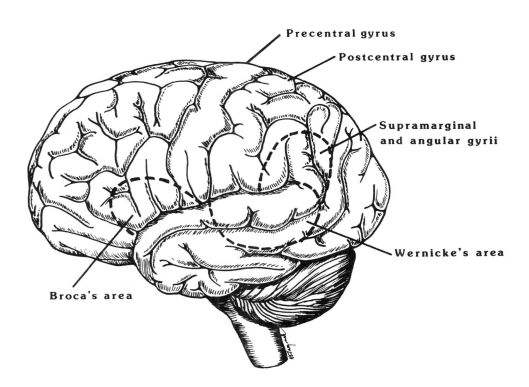

Precentral gyrus

Postcentral gyrus

Supramarginal
and angular gyrii

Wernicke's area

Broca's area

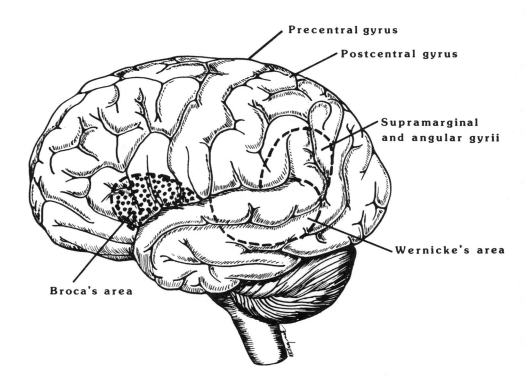

Precentral gyrus

Postcentral gyrus

Supramarginal
and angular gyrii

Wernicke's area

Broca's area

Speech/oral apraxia compatible with a left lateral inferior frontal lobe lesion involving Broca's area.

Discussion The history and pathogenesis of this patient's motor speech findings were consistent with stroke. In the absence of a history of hypertension, however, the etiology was rather unclear. A cardiovascular problem was considered. Approximately two months after the present hospitalization, the patient suffered another left-side CVA, which rendered her globally aphasic. Again, the etiology was unclear. However, ultrasound and cardiac evaluation subsequently revealed an atrial myxoma, which was removed surgically. The etiology of her vascular events therefore was considered cardioembolic in origin.

In severe cases of apraxia of speech the motor planning deficit may be so severe that the patient may be unable to initiate phonation on request, even though vestigial laryngeal function, including coughing and throat clearing, remain intact. The deficit may also influence swallowing, in which the patient has difficulty "programming" the oral speech musculature to move food posteriorly. Unilateral facial and lingual weakness, secondary to contralateral corticobulbar tract involvement, may exacerbate this process.

This patient's apraxia of speech and coexistant neuromuscular signs involving the right face, tongue, arm, and leg can be explained on the basis of involvement of the distal anterior branches of the left middle cerebral artery. Such damage frequently impairs functioning of Brodmann's area 44 as well as the majority of the precentral gyrus of the left cerebral hemisphere. Although we inferred such involvements were responsible for the symptoms in our patient, we initially could not substantiate our suspicions since CT and EEG findings were "normal." On her second admission, however, CT scan revealed a left hemispheric infarct.

The patient was discharged from initial admission on 50 mg of dipyridamole (Persantine) 3 times a day, and was seen for outpatient speech therapy. Her apraxia of speech resolved almost completely and she was left with only mild right face and tongue weakness. Unfortunately, the second stroke exacerbated the residual findings and left her with a dense global aphasia as well as right-side hemiplegia. At the time of this report, the patient was being seen for outpatient therapy.

57-Year-Old Female with Headache and Language Disturbance

History

This healthy 57-year-old female was preparing to bake a cake, when she developed a throbbing frontal headache. Two aspirins relieved the symptoms for about an hour; however, the pain soon recurred. Because she appeared unsteady on her feet, and had difficulty reading the baking instructions, her husband drove her to the clinic for an evaluation. He had suffered a very mild stroke a year earlier, and was concerned that his wife's symptoms might be related to a stroke. She was admitted to hospital for testing.

Examination

The patient was alert throughout the testing; however, she exhibited moderate inability to follow audible or written one- and two-step commands. The words she used in response to most questions were "yes" and "no;" these utterances were effortful. Gait was unsteady with a slight drift to the right side. However, there was no evidence of hemiparesis on a more complete limb examination.

Alternate motion rates of the fingers and hand on the right side were slower than normal, and slightly irregular. Tendon reflexes were unremarkable, although there was a question of a Babinski on the right. No bruits were heard in the neck, and x-rays and physical examination of the chest were normal. Cranial nerve functions were normal.

EXTENSION OF THE GREAT TOE W/ FANNING OF THE OTHER TOES ON STIMULATION OF THE SOLE OF THE FOOT ; MAY BE INDICATIVE OF A LESION INVOLVING THE PYRAMIDAL TRACT.

CT scan revealed areas of decreased density in the left temporal-parietal zones, including the supramarginal and angular gyrii. Cerebral angiography illustrated marked stenosis of the internal carotid artery and multiple middle cerebral artery branch occlusions on the left.

Expressive speech and language were markedly dysfluent. Along with "yes" "no" utterances, certain automatic phrases like: "I love you," "who's there?" "how are you?" and "fine, thank you" were articulated normally and spontaneously in response to questions. The patient was able to imitate virtually all single words, even those containing multiple syllables, effortlessly and without error. However, writing spontaneously and to dictation was ungrammatical, and plagued by word selection and recall errors.

Auditory and visual comprehension deficits were severe; one- and two-step commands were errored more than 90 percent of the time. Auditory memory span was limited to two words or digits; word fluency could not be assessed, as the patient remained silent during this phase of testing. Prompts to elicit word fluency capability were unsuccessful. Naming objects and demonstrating their functions were significantly impaired. There were no apparent signs of volitional oral motor control deficits.

Salient symptoms/signs	Test results	Impressions

This worksheet is to be used for recording relevant diagnostic observations. The blank illustration is to be used for identifying and sketching the suspected site of lesion(s). These steps should be completed prior to turning to the Impressions and illustrated site of lesion.

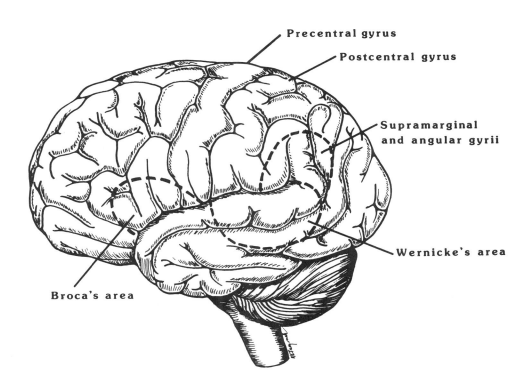

Precentral gyrus

Postcentral gyrus

Supramarginal
and angular gyrii

Wernicke's area

Broca's area

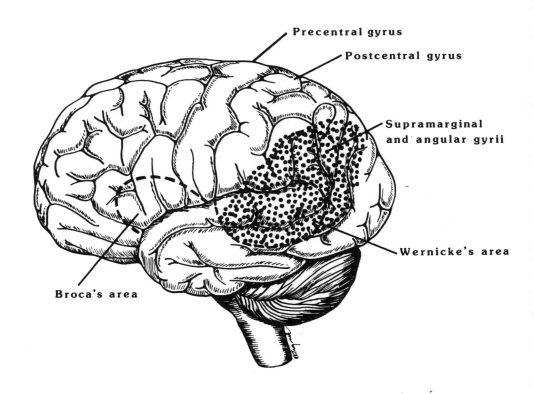

Precentral gyrus

Postcentral gyrus

Supramarginal
and angular gyrii

Wernicke's area

Broca's area

Impressions   Aphasia due to infarction of the left cerebral hemisphere; middle cerebral artery distribution.

Discussion   Our patient's language deficit suggests damage to the components of the central language processor in the left hemisphere. Her language and speech symptoms are characteristic of aphasia. Her impaired limb alternate motion rate, mild gait abnormalities, and Babinski sign are manifestations of a mild motor system disturbance.

It is well understood that the zones of language processing receive their blood supply from the pre-Rolandic and middle temporal branches of the middle cerebral artery. Cerebral angiography revealed stenosis of the main trunk of the left internal carotid artery, as well as multiple occlusions of its distal middle cerebral artery branches. Aphasia is a common sequela to such arterial involvements. Usually, an associated right hemiparesis, indicative of a lesion in the left pyramidal system, also prevails. This was not so in our case.

When aphasia occurs without hemiparesis, one can postulate that the pyramidal tract on the involved side has been spared. Slight or minor contralateral motor signs, as in our patient, are typically due to edema and tend to improve rather rapidly. Because of the proximity of the postcentral gyrus to the lesion in aphasia patients, contralateral sensory impairments, including involvement of the face, are not uncommon. In our patient, the sensory strip and tracts were apparently spared or recovered.

An infarct is an area of necrosis in a tissue owing to obstruction in its blood supply. Angiography and CT scan substantiated our diagnosis of cerebral infarction. At the time of this report, the patient was receiving speech-language therapy; her prognosis for improvement remained guarded.

60-Year-Old Female with Writer's Cramp and Voice Symptoms

History   This 60-year-old, right-handed female nursing instructor was referred to speech pathology for further evaluation of phonatory and laryngeal function subsequent to a normal otolaryngologic examination two weeks before being seen. Eighteen years earlier, she had been diagnosed by a neurologist as having intermittent writer's cramp. At that time, the symptoms were not believed to be significant enough to either the patient or the examiner to warrant medical therapy. She was taking medication for menopausal symptoms and chronic mild hypothyroidism. She was otherwise healthy. There was no history of marital or psychoemotional discord.

Examination   The patient was pleasant, attentive, well-kempt, but somewhat anxious on examination. Cranial nerves V (motor and sensory), VII, and IX through XII were functioning within normal limits. There were no pathologic reflexes. A slight Class III malocclusion (prognathia) was evident that resulted in minimal distortion of sibilant sounds but did not impair speech intelligibility. The remainder of the findings were confined to laryngeal/phonatory function.

Conversational speech was characterized by moderate strain-strangled quality with fleeting adductory voice arrest. Vowel prolongation was characterized by intermittent islands of regular changes in volume estimated to be between 6 and 8 Hz, without voice arrests. Acoustic analysis further delineated the perceptual phonatory signs. Laryngeal endoscopy with video stroboscopy revealed intermittent tremulous movements of the larynx on vowel prolongation, these movements being absent at rest. Subsequent neurologic reevaluation was within normal limits; writer's cramp was not observed nor could it be elicited.

Salient symptoms/signs	Test results	Impressions

This worksheet is to be used for recording relevant diagnostic observations. The blank illustration is to be used for identifying and sketching the suspected site of lesion(s). These steps should be completed prior to turning to the Impressions and illustrated site of lesion.

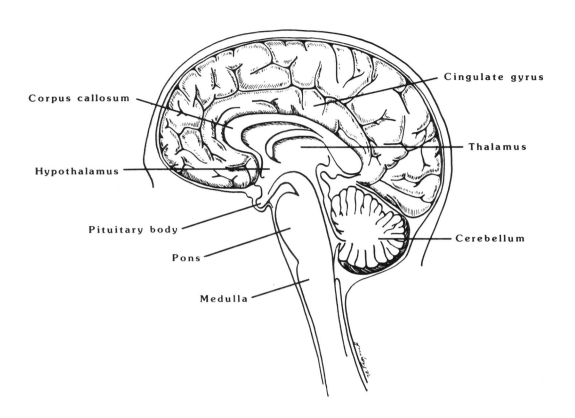

Corpus callosum

Cingulate gyrus

Thalamus

Hypothalamus

Pituitary body

Cerebellum

Pons

Medulla

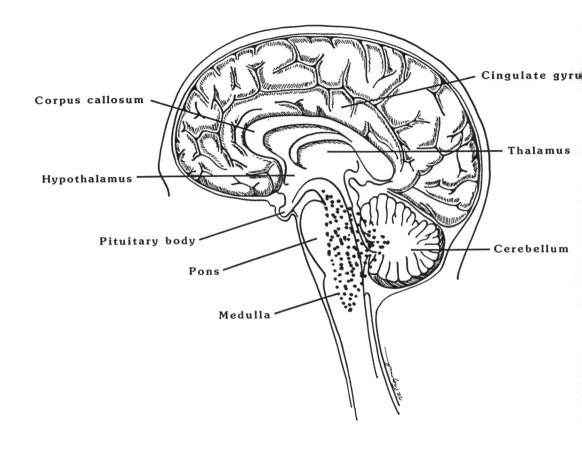

Corpus callosum

Hypothalamus

Pituitary body

Pons

Medulla

Cingulate gyru

Thalamus

Cerebellum

Impressions   Early mild spastic (spasmodic) dysphonia or comparable essential voice tremor in a patient with a history of chronic intermittent focal dystonia—writer's cramp.

Discussion   It is generally the consensus among those who study movement disorders that the majority of patients who present with signs of spasmodic dysphonia actually have a focal laryngeal dystonia. It should be noted, however, that in some patients the spasmodic dysphonia represents psychopathology rather than a focal movement disorder. The presence of voice arrest *and* tremor generally points to a neurogenic cause. Patients with segmental dystonia (that is, primary involvement in one body part) eventually develop dystonic features in other parts of the body, as in this patient's case. To date, our patient's symptoms and signs have been confined to the right upper extremity and her larynx. She does not view them as disabling and, therefore, has not sought therapy. Because her mild dysphonic symptoms consisting principally of tremor may evolve into a more widespread and severe movement disorder, she continues to be followed in speech pathology and neurology. At this time, the preponderance of research would point to brainstem involvement for both voice tremor and laryngeal dystonia.

40-Year-Old Female with Neck Pain, Head Movements, and Speech Disturbance

History A 40-year-old housewife with an unremarkable medical background complained of a gradual onset of pain in the right neck accompanied by an uncontrolled rotation of the head to the right, which was most evident while sitting. The situation caused her to have considerable difficulty while reading, watching television, and attempting to maintain eye contact with those to whom she was speaking. She believed that the changes in her speech, which had been called to her attention by her husband, were associated with the positioning of her head.

Examination With the patient in the sitting position, her head gradually rotated to the right and became partially dorsiflexed. She was unable to change this posture in the seated position, but could modify it somewhat, but incompletely when standing. The sternocleidomastoid and trapezius muscles on the left were mildly hypertrophied and hypertonic. Occasional clonic spasms of the platysma on the left, with concurrent depression of the left lower face, were also noted.

Phonation in conversational speech was characterized by a harsh voice quality, periods of breathiness, variations in loudness, and mon-opitch. On vowel prolongation, the loudness variations were more noticeable and occasional voice arrests evident. Articulation was mildly imprecise due to distortion of consonant sounds. Oral diadochokinetic and sequential motion rates were mildly irregular and slow. Respiration for speech appeared somewhat effortful. The remainder of the examination was unremarkable, as was the routine psychiatric screening examination.

Salient symptoms/signs	Test results	Impressions

This worksheet is to be used for recording relevant diagnostic observations. The blank illustration is to be used for identifying and sketching the suspected site of lesion(s). These steps should be completed prior to turning to the Impressions and illustrated site of lesion.

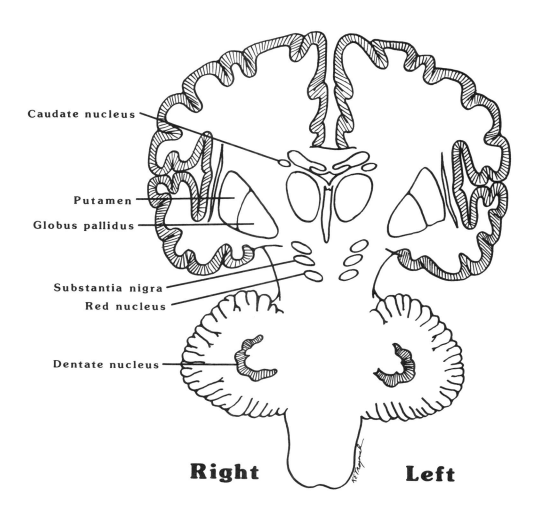

Caudate nucleus

Putamen

Globus pallidus

Substantia nigra

Red nucleus

Dentate nucleus

Right

Left

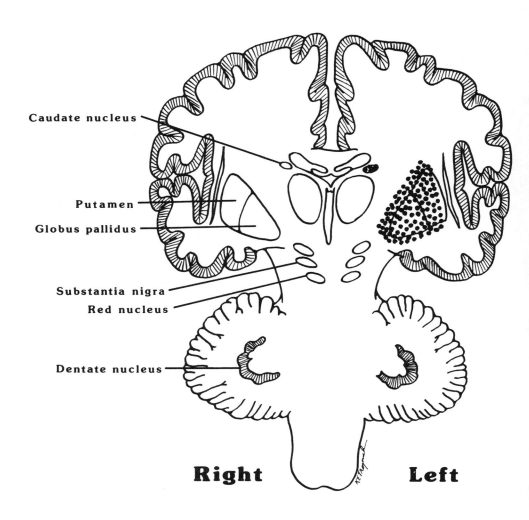

Caudate nucleus

Putamen

Globus pallidus

Substantia nigra
Red nucleus

Dentate nucleus

Right　　　　**Left**

Impressions   Hyperkinetic (slow) dysarthria; dystonia.

Discussion   The XIth cranial nerve innervates the sternocleidomastoid and trapezius muscles. It is represented primarily in an uncrossed fashion, on a supranuclear basis. A lesion involving the globus pallidus and striatum will result in an increased tone and cocontraction of agonist and antagonist muscles, causing the head to rotate to the side opposite the lesion.

The abnormal posturing of the head and neck, as in this case of spasmodic torticollis, a form of dystonia, disturbs the relationship among intrinsic and extrinsic laryngeal muscles as well as the entire vocal tract. The results of this posture is abnormal phonation.

Mild articulatory imprecision could be due to dystonic movements of the peri- and intraoral musculature persistent in conversational speech, clonic spasms of the inframandibular musculature, or both. The respiratory signs could be due to the hypertonicity of the sterno-cleidomastoid and trapezius muscles, which are sometimes considered accessory muscles of respiration.

Spasmodic torticollis is frequently intractable and may be an early sign of a more widespread dystonia. Currently the standard for care for this movement disorder is recurrent botulinum toxin injections into the affected sternocleidomastoid muscle. Some patients with spasmodic torticollis may experience some relief with the anticholinergic agents or diazepam (Valium). Neurectomy has been less successful because of the number of muscles involved.

38-Year-Old Female with a Positive Familial History Has Limb, Trunk, and Speech Musculature Incoordination

History   For approximately three years, a 38-year-old housewife experienced slight incoordination of gait and upper limb activities, which did not interfere significantly with her household chores or other responsibilities. Medical evaluations throughout this period of time were inconclusive as to the cause of her difficulties, and no specific recommendations were made.

During the fourth year of her motor difficulties, she experienced a marked increase in incoordination of gait and upper limb activities. She also complained of trembling of her hands, which occurred only when she moved her arms intentionally, and problems with tongue and lip control, which interfered slightly with speech intelligibility. She was referred for neurologic and speech-language evaluations.

Examination   A familial history of similar motor difficulties was uncovered in the paternal lineage; however, her father did not himself experience these signs and symptoms.

Gait was reeling, unsteady and wide based with a tendency to teeter to the right. Finger-to-nose and heel-to-knee tasks were incoordinated and off target, and hand and arm movements were characterized by terminal intention tremors, which subsided at rest; these signs were more pronounced on the right side. Limb musculature was mildly hypotonic and hyporeflexive on the left side of the body and moderately so on the right. Alternate motion rates of the hands were slow and irregular.

The tongue was hypotonic. Tongue wiggling and other nonspeech movements were considered incoordinated and slow. Articulation was found to be mild to moderately imprecise and slow.

Voice was characterized by sudden outbursts of loudness and pitch alterations, and duration of phonation was moderately reduced. Frequently, more than one breath was required to complete a simple sentence. Vowel prolongations sounded mildly harsh and tremulous. Labial and lingual alternate and sequential motion rates were mildly slow, imprecise, and moderately dysrhythmic.

Salient symptoms/signs	Test results	Impressions

This worksheet is to be used for recording relevant diagnostic observations. The blank illustration is to be used for identifying and sketching the suspected site of lesion(s). These steps should be completed prior to turning to the Impressions and illustrated site of lesion.

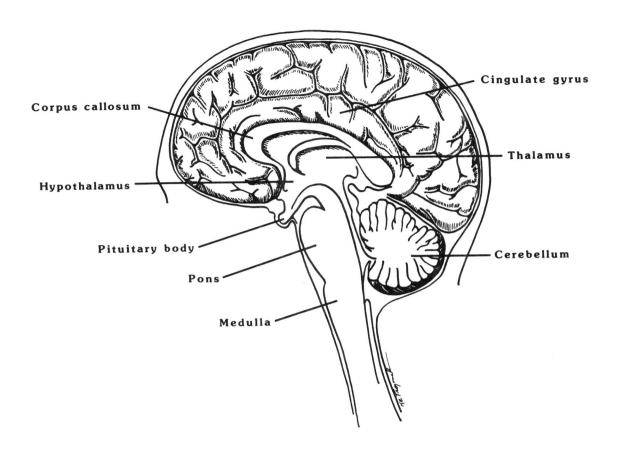

Corpus callosum

Cingulate gyrus

Hypothalamus

Thalamus

Pituitary body

Cerebellum

Pons

Medulla

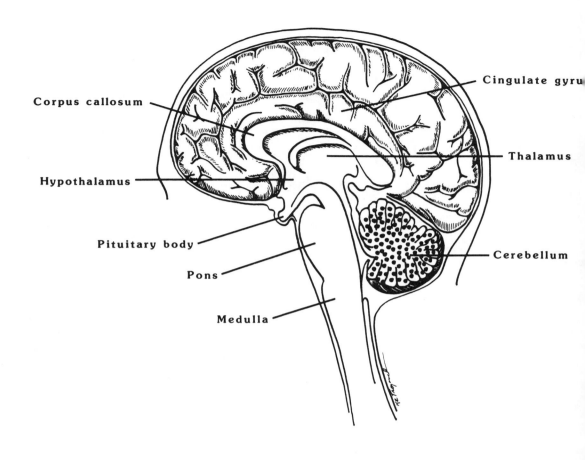

Corpus callosum

Cingulate gyru

Thalamus

Hypothalamus

Pituitary body

Pons

Cerebellum

Medulla

Impressions   Ataxic dysarthria and generalized dyssynergia due to hereditary cerebellar degeneration.

Discussion   This patient exhibited signs of cerebellar degeneration, which proved to be of familial origin. Gait ataxia results from damage to the vermis of the cerebellum where impulses normally pass via the fastigial nuclei to the vestibular nuclei to help regulate posture and balance.

It is also known that lesions of the flocculonodular lobe of the cerebellum may cause trunk ataxia, since this area functions to orient the body in space. Teetering to the right suggests that involvement of these areas may be more pronounced on the right half of the cerebellum than on the left side.

Dysmetrias (past-pointing phenomena) are characterized by inability to estimate accurately ranges of voluntary movements. For example, on a finger-to-nose task, the finger shoots past the nose onto the cheek. Lesions of the dentate nuclei in the cerebellar hemispheres may result in dysmetrias, as well as the types of intention tremors and alternate motion rate irregularities seen in this case.

Normally, impulses from the motor and premotor strips of the cortex are relayed via the pontocerebellar tracts to the dentate nuclei. These nuclei, in turn, send impulses through the superior cerebellar penduncles to the red nucleus and thalamus and thence back to the motor strips, forming a closed "feedback" circuit or "servomechanism" between the cerebral cortex and cerebellum. These interconnections play an important role in regulating the rhythm, speed, force, and range of muscular contractions.

Ataxic dysarthria most often results from bilateral cerebellar degeneration or lesions involving the vermis. The affected speech muscles move slowly, and their timing, range and force of contractions are incoordinated and imprecise; they also tend to be hypotonic and flabby. Articulation is imprecise and speech sounds slurred, as movements of the lips and tongue are variably slow, irregular, and excessive.

Phonation is characterized by periodic outbursts of loudness and pitch changes, owing to the irregularity of the speed, amplitude, and force of vocal fold vibrations. Sometimes a trembling of the entire larynx occurs, causing tremorlike quality of the voice. Involvement of the respiratory musculature and resultant irregularity of breathing may cause reduced length of phrases, excess loudness, inappropriate pitch variations, and explosive patterns of articulation.

38-Year-Old Male with Deterioration of Speech, Language, and Right Side Control

History   When she returned from a grocery store, the wife of a 38-year-old male found him lying on the floor unconscious. She immediately called their family physician and an ambulance was summoned to take him to the hospital. Enroute he regained consciousness, but did not verbally respond or answer questions posed by the emergency medical team or his wife, though he appeared to understand what they were asking of him.

At the admission desk, the wife divulged that for the past two months, the patient had been experiencing progressive weakness and numbness on the entire right side of his body. Both thought that his symptoms were due to muscle strain incurred during their weekly racquetball games, and therefore did not consult their physician.

Examination   During testing, the patient appeared moderately depressed, but alert and cooperative. He was able to sit up on the examining table without assistance, though he favored his left side. Moderate to severe hemiparesis and an associated positive Babinski sign were evident on the right side. No other bodily signs were noted. With the exceptions of mild to moderate central facial and tongue weakness on the right side, the speech mechanism was neuromuscularly intact. Cerebral angiography and CT scan revealed a large subdural mass located over the left frontal and parietal regions.

The patient's answers to questions about his medical history, job as a machinist, and family life were markedly hesitant, and limited almost exclusively to one- or two-word utterances. His telegraphic-type answers, however, were judged to be related to the questions asked. For example, when asked whether he preferred to read or watch TV during his spare time, he replied, "read." When asked whether he read novels, nonfiction, or magazines, he replied, "Oh dear; uh—books."

His spontaneous speech was moderately nonfluent, slow, and laborious. He did not use inflections to signal an interrogative; most utterances were amelodic. Functor words such as "to," "and," and "the" were not used, thereby rendering his speech telegraphic and agrammatical. Multiple articulation errors were noted, many of which were considered anticipatory, such as "lipow" for "pillow."

His auditory comprehension was much better than his speech output, but not normal. He could repeat no more than three digits in a forward order, or two digits in reverse order. When asked complex questions like "What day comes after Tuesday?" he responded, "no—no!" He could name the days of the week in correct order. He repeated words and sentences with less dysfluency, agrammatism, and articulatory difficulty than during spontaneous speech.

Because of the paretic preferred right upper extremity, he used his left hand to write. With the exception of obvious orthographic changes associated with writing with the nonpreferred hand, many written errors mirrored his spoken ones; that is, there were frequent letter substitutions and transpositions within words.

Salient symptoms/signs	Test results	Impressions

This worksheet is to be used for recording relevant diagnostic observations. The blank illustration is to be used for identifying and sketching the suspected site of lesion(s). These steps should be completed prior to turning to the Impressions and illustrated site of lesion.

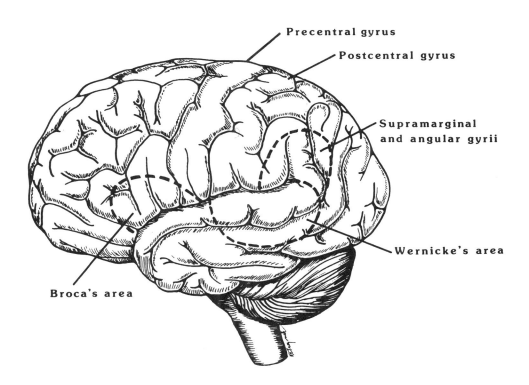

Precentral gyrus

Postcentral gyrus

Supramarginal
and angular gyrii

Wernicke's area

Broca's area

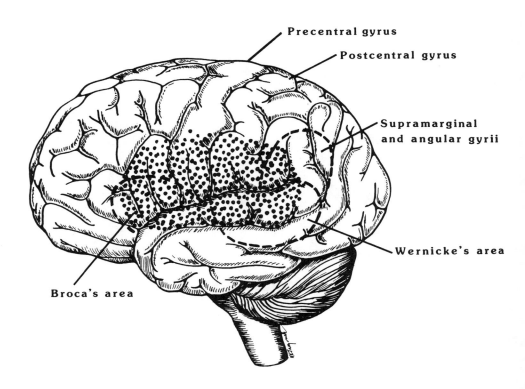

Precentral gyrus

Postcentral gyrus

Supramarginal
and angular gyrii

Wernicke's area

Broca's area

Impressions Apraxia of speech and aphasia due to a left hemisphere subdural mass.

Discussion Three days after admission to hospital, the patient underwent surgical evacuation of a moderately large abscess located over the left frontal and parietal areas. Shortly thereafter the neurological deficits cleared to a large extent. The central facial (lower two-thirds of the face) and tongue weakness on the right side are consistent with left corticobulbar tract impairment. Most patients with apraxia of speech exhibit these associated motor signs.

The speech of individuals with apraxia of speech (roughly synonymous with what has been called Broca's or nonfluent aphasia) may be classified as halting, labored, ungrammatical, monotonous, and inarticulate. In an acute form, the patient may be mute.

Auditory and visual comprehension deficits (language impairments) are likely to be detected in all patients with apraxia of speech. These problems, however, are usually not as severe as the motor planning deficit, and are typically ascribed to postcentral sulcus involvement, as in this patient. It is more often the rule than the exception that apraxia of speech and aphasia coexist and contribute to the communicative signs.

Speech therapy was directed toward improving the patient's prosodic, articulatory, and language difficulties. With three weeks of intensive therapy, the patient had improved marginally.

24-Year-Old Male with Closed Head Injury and Language Disturbance

History A 24-year-old male high school teacher was driving home from a party, at which he consumed an excessive amount of alcohol, when he was involved in a head-on collision with another automobile. At the scene of the accident, he was unconscious and unresponsive to routine stimulus testing by the emergency team. A deep 20 x 5 cm frontal bone laceration and a 7 x 3 cm right temporal bone laceration were detected. No palpable skull fractures were evident, however. The patient was rushed to hospital for further examination and care.

Examination The patient was comatose at admission to hospital, with a Glasgow Coma Scale score of 8. He withdrew from painful stimuli administered on the right side of his body, and was decorticate on the left. Deep tendon reflexes could not be evoked, and an equivocal Babinski sign was noted on the left. His eyes remained closed during testing, except when he was pinched. He was unable to converse with the attending physician. CT scan revealed bleeding in the lateral and third ventricles, with no discernible mass effect or shift. A temporal lobe hemorrhage was also evident on the right.

Two days postadmission, a left frontal subarachnoid intracranial pressure monitor was placed. On the first postoperative day, he was more responsive to painful stimuli and was able to move all extremities. Due to his increased response to test stimuli and coherence, he was rated at 12 on the Glasgow Coma Scale.

Two days later speech-language assessment revealed that the patient was oriented to person, family and staff, but disoriented to date, place and situation. He could follow one- and two-step commands consistently; however, his short and long term memory were significantly impaired. Frequent prompts were required to induce attending behaviors, and he was unable to go through daily schedules without confusion. Copying simple block or pegboard designs, reproducing pictures, drawing a person or house, and matching geometric shapes were significantly impaired.

He was easily agitated, distracted, and confused by external stimuli. He frequently responded appropriately with prompting and redirection. Speech was articulate and fluent; language use was adequate at basic conversational levels. However, he demonstrated difficulty integrating and organizing more complex and lengthy spoken and written stimuli. Metaphors and idioms were particularly difficult for him to analyze. Poor attention span and memory made answering questions about a novel's storyline virtually impossible. Auditory comprehension of less complex stimuli, however, was relatively well preserved. Reading comprehension was mildly impaired.

Salient symptoms/signs	Test results	Impressions

This worksheet is to be used for recording relevant diagnostic observations. The blank illustration is to be used for identifying and sketching the suspected site of lesion(s). These steps should be completed prior to turning to the Impressions and illustrated site of lesion.

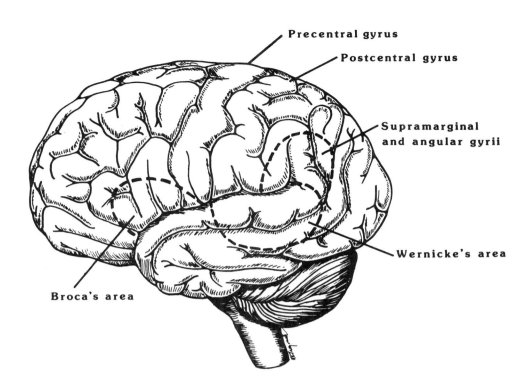

Precentral gyrus

Postcentral gyrus

Supramarginal
and angular gyrii

Wernicke's area

Broca's area

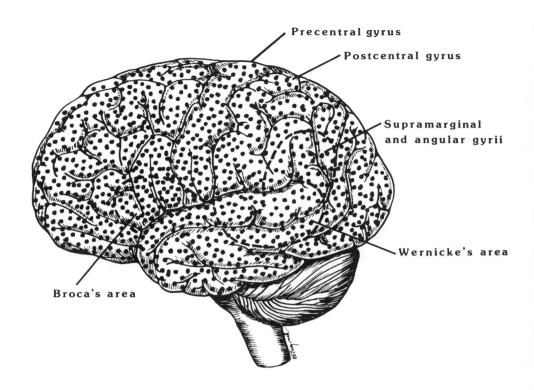

Precentral gyrus

Postcentral gyrus

Supramarginal
and angular gyrii

Wernicke's area

Broca's area

Impressions　Language of confusion due to closed head injury.

Discussion　Head injury frequently results in communication deficits. The type of deficit varies depending upon the degree and site of injury. Because the effects of a head injury usually vary during the different stages of recovery, communication and other difficulties also vary. In this patient the communicative disturbances following head trauma are consistent with what has been called *confused language*. The term is used to help distinguish the deficit from focal communicative disorders such as aphasia. However, aphasic signs are frequently embedded within the language of confusion. With time and therapy, the patient is typically left with a broad, less focal impairment.

The Glasgow Coma Scale was developed to establish universal means of defining coma. It relies on three basic measures assessed across a 15-point scale: (1) eye opening; (2) motor response; and (3) verbal ability. For example: "Eyes open volitionally and spontaneously" receives a score of 4, and "eyes unable to be open" a score of 1. "Relatively normal conversational speech and language responses" receives a score of 5, and "makes no noise" a score of 1. Over 90 percent of those who score 8 or less are in coma, as was this patient. Those scoring above 8 may have sustained minor to moderate brain injury, but are not in coma.

With the exception of mild ataxic gait, implicating the cerebellar system, our patient's original sensorimotor deficits resolved nicely in the course of his recovery. Speech-language intervention began approximately one month postinjury with focus on improving: (1) selective attention skills; (2) memory, both short and long term; (3) word retrieval, storage and symbolic organization of simple as well as complex linguistic material; (4) sequential organization, reasoning, and problem-solving abilities; and (5) reading comprehension and written expression.

Four months later, the patient's problem-solving and reasoning abilities remained concrete. Reading comprehension had improved, but remained depressed. Grammatical and spelling errors continue to plague the patient's written work. Vague and disorganized thought patterns compounded such errors, rendering his written expression significantly impaired. Abstract stimuli continued to be more difficult to process than concrete material. He was able to make his needs known verbally, and situational language use was adequate.

31-Year-Old Female with Intermittent Numbness, Double Vision, Urinary Incontinence, and Speech Disturbance

History A 31-year-old saleswoman reported to her physician that over the course of one year she had been experiencing numbness of her hands, double vision, difficulty tying her shoes and performing other fine manual activities, slight tremor of the arms, urinary incontinence, and slurred speech. She remarked that the reason she had waited so long before requesting evaluation was that in the past these difficulties would remit spontaneously. Presently they seemed to linger and were more disabling.

Examination The patient used age appropriate language, and was attentive and cooperative throughout testing. The following salient signs and symptoms were identified: (1) minimal loss of visual acuity in the right eye, with associated pain in that eye when gazing at a moving object; (2) pallor of both optic discs; (3) broad-based and incoordinated gait; (4) generalized hyperreflexia and moderate loss of joint position and vibration sense in all four extremities; (5) inability to perform normally fine skilled movements of the hands or feet; (6) intention tremor in both arms; (7) overshooting or misjudging the degree of movement necessary to perform finger-to-nose, heel-to-knee, and reaching tasks; (8) moderate weakness, paresis, and hypertonicity of all four limbs; (9) bilateral Babinski signs; (10) slow and dysrhythmic alternating motion rates of the hands; (11) exaggerated gag and associated orofacial reflexes; (12) reduced range and speed of movement of the tongue and lips, without evidence of atrophy or fasciculations; (13) vocal harshness; (14) impaired speech emphasis, characterized by excessive and inappropriate rate, phrasing, loudness, and pitch control; (15) distorted articulation; (16) variable hypernasality; and (17) slow and dysrhythmic lingual and labial alternate motion rates.

Hot baths precipitated double vision, urinary incontinence, and increased difficulty with fine motor skill tasks. Visual evoked response testing proved inconclusive; however, brainstem auditory evoked responses were abnormal. Cerebrospinal fluid analysis revealed a mildly increased level of gamma globulin.

Salient symptoms/signs	Test results	Impressions

This worksheet is to be used for recording relevant diagnostic observations. The blank illustration is to be used for identifying and sketching the suspected site of lesion(s). These steps should be completed prior to turning to the Impressions and illustrated site of lesion.

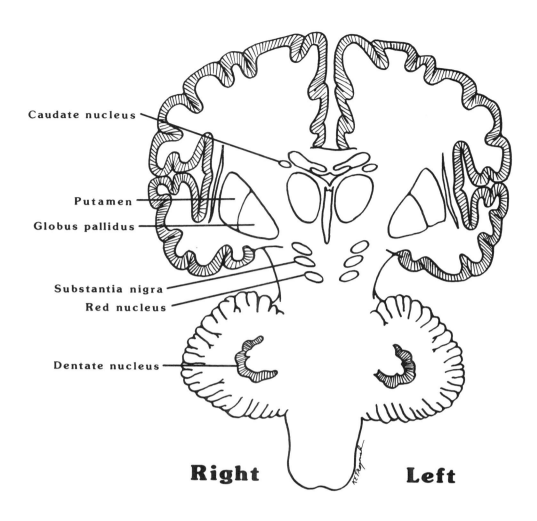

Caudate nucleus

Putamen

Globus pallidus

Substantia nigra

Red nucleus

Dentate nucleus

Right

Left

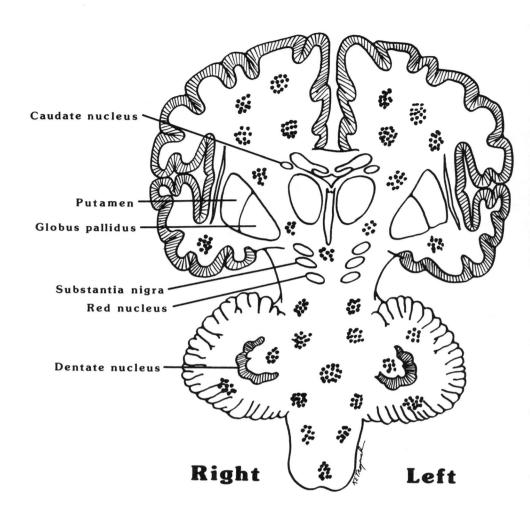

Caudate nucleus

Putamen

Globus pallidus

Substantia nigra

Red nucleus

Dentate nucleus

Right

Left

Impressions   Mixed ataxic-spastic dysarthria, caused by multiple sclerosis.

Discussion   Generally occuring during the third and fourth decades of life, multiple sclerosis (MS) is a central nervous system disease. It primarily affects the fibers of the pyramidal system as they course through the brain, brainstem, spinal cord, and cerebellum. The involvement of myelin (demyelinization) varies from slight swelling to complete degeneration.

The nature of this disease is such that new plaques may form at any time over the course of many years, and in any area within the white matter of the central nervous system (CNS). In the initial stage of the disease, exacerbations and remissions of symptoms are very common. As plaque formation increases, the clinical picture usually becomes more severe and prolonged. An exacerbation of a symptom may represent: (1) a new plaque; (2) an enlargement of an old plaque; and (3) a physiologic reaction to heat, body, or emotional stress.

This patient exhibited many of the classic signs and symptoms of MS, including difficulties with vision and urinary incontinence. The ataxic gait, intention tremors, and incoordinated limb performances are characteristic of cerebellar involvement. The articulatory imprecision, prosodic insufficiencies and dysrhythmic alternate motion rates illustrated the effects of such involvement on the timing and coordination of speech.

Co-occuring with the ataxic signs were an assortment of findings that implicated the pyramidal system. These included exaggerated reflexes, Babinski signs, and slowness, weakness, paresis, and hypertonicity. The articulatory imprecision was considered secondary to slow rate and weak tongue movements, while the harsh voice quality and hypernasality indicated involvement of the lingual, velopharyngeal, and laryngeal musculature.

When the diagnosticians can demonstrate the presence of multiple lesions in the CNS, as evidenced by the neurologic deficits and history of the patient, MS may be considered a possible cause, especially if there has been a relapsing and remitting course of symptoms.

Certain laboratory tests help, either by producing evidence of scattered plaque formation, or providing other conclusive diagnostic data. It is known that heat as experienced in a warm bath may either exacerbate symptoms of MS, or precipitate new ones. Auditory evoked response audiometry may suggest plaque formation throughout the brainstem. The increased gamma globulin count is yet another finding that helps corroborate the diagnosis.

Steroids were prescribed to help shorten the acute attacks, but were discontinued one month later. The efficacy of such medication in the treatment of MS still remains undetermined. Although at the time of this report our patient's double vision was not debilitating, some patients find relief from this condition by wearing an eye patch. Baclofen mildly modified the limb hypertonicity. Medications, along with bladder training and regular dieting, improved the urinary problems.

Speech therapy focused on improving rate, phrasing, and articulatory proficiency. Exercises designed to improve the strength, tone, and range of movement of the tongue and lips were incorporated along with speech drills. Since laryngeal and velopharyngeal breakdowns secondary to neuromuscular impairments are not typically amenable to speech intervention techniques, an otolaryngologist and prosthodontist were consulted to determine if the hypernasality might be improved by pharyngoplasty or a palatal-lift prosthesis. Neither had been attempted with our patient at the time of this report.

16-Year-Old Female with Nasal Emission

History This 16-year-old female was referred by her mother for evaluation of speech and a "buzzing" sound from her nose apparent when the patient played the clarinet. This symptom had developed gradually in the three to four weeks before being seen and was noted only when the youth played her instrument. In an attempt to alleviate the symptoms, she had tried wearing nose plugs or placing cotton in her nose when playing. However, because this drew unwanted attention, she chose not to implement these facilitating techniques.

There were no reported changes in speech or language, nor were there cognitive complaints. There were no changes in vision, handwriting, hearing, or gait. As an active, rather intense student, she was maintaining an "A" average during her junior year in high school.

Her prior medical history was significant for familial neurofibromatosis. She had been seen previously in ophthalmology for neurofibroma of both irises and dermatology for discussion of removal of two skin neurofibromas. Previous audiometric and pediatric neurologic evaluations had been well within normal limits.

Examination Examination revealed a pleasant, attractive, straightforward patient who looked her age. Examination of the oral mechanism revealed functally normal cranial nerves V (motor and sensory), VII, XI, and XII. The jaw jerk was mildly brisk. The pharyngeal reflex was sluggish but symmetrical, as were movements of the velum during production of vowels. The structural integrity of the speech mechanism was sound for speech production.

Conversational speech and production of non-nasal sequences revealed mild hypernasality with islands of nasal emission that improved with anterior occlusion of the nares. Protracted effortful speech did not result in deterioration in quality or speech precision. Laryngeal structure and function were normal on endoscopic examination, although voice quality was mildly breathy. Articulation, respiration, and the prosodic elements of speech were well within normal limits. There were no language or cognitive signs.

Salient symptoms/signs	Test results	Impressions

This worksheet is to be used for recording relevant diagnostic observations. The blank illustration is to be used for identifying and sketching the suspected site of lesion(s). These steps should be completed prior to turning to the Impressions and illustrated site of lesion.

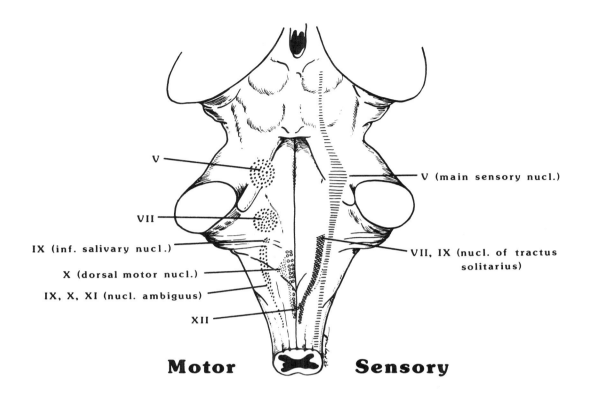

Motor   **Sensory**

V

VII

IX (inf. salivary nucl.)

X (dorsal motor nucl.)

IX, X, XI (nucl. ambiguus)

XII

V (main sensory nucl.)

VII, IX (nucl. of tractus solitarius)

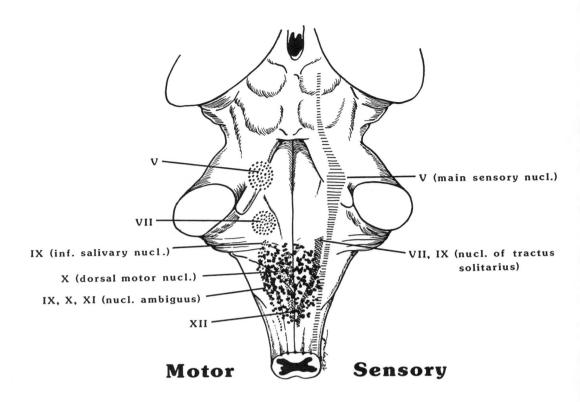

V

V (main sensory nucl.)

VII

IX (inf. salivary nucl.)

X (dorsal motor nucl.)

IX, X, XI (nucl. ambiguus)

XII

VII, IX (nucl. of tractus
solitarius)

Motor　　　**Sensory**

Impressions   Mild flaccid dysarthria manifested principally by velopharyngeal incompetence in a patient with known neurofibromatosis.

Discussion   Given the patient's history and concern for brainstem lesion, the patient was referred to pediatric neurology with a recommendation for MRI of the head, particularly the posterior fossa and brainstem. The results of this study revealed a large high-density lesion in the lower medulla in the region of the IX and X nerve nuclei, bilaterally felt to be consistent with a neurofibroma. These nerves innervate the velopharynx and larynx.

Von Recklinghausen neurofibromatosis is a relatively rare heredofamilial disease that may affect the skin, nervous system, and other organs of the body. The clinician is alerted to the disorder by the presence of multiple circumscribed areas of skin pigmentation (café au lait spots) frequently accompanied by dermal and/or neural tumors, which are generally benign. The II, V, and VIII cranial nerves are particularly subject to neurofibromatous changes with resultant visual, facial/masticatory, and auditory motor and sensory symptoms and signs. Brain involvement may result in cognitive impairment and seizures in some patients. In our patient, involvement of the nucleus ambiguus directly, as a result of mass effect from the tumor or both, was believed to be responsible for the resonatory signs. The patient not showing signs of more widespread involvement of the brainstem (including laryngeal function) may have been from slow growth of the tumor and concurrent adaptation of the neural circuitry in that area. Many neurofibromas are amenable to excision although there is a tendency for recurrence. Radiation or chemotherapy is not indicated in the treatment of the disease.

The symptoms in our patient were rather minimal; therefore, it was the consensus that she should be followed with periodic clinical reevaluation and MRI rather than undergoing a neurosurgical procedure. We suggested a palatal lift appliance to improve intraoral breath pressure while playing the clarinet. The youth was not interested in the recommendation.

50-Year-Old Hypertensive Female with Speech Disturbance

History After the death of her son, a 50-year-old hypertensive housewife went into a severe state of depression, with chronic episodes of crying and remorse that lingered for three years. One day she became dizzy and felt weak. She also stated that she felt "giddy" and that her speech sounded slurred and stutterlike. Over the course of the next week, the weakness persisted while her speech may have worsened. She began to drool and regurgitate liquids through the nose, and she laughed and cried without provocation.

Examination Reflexes were brisk bilaterally. There were no sensory findings. Bilateral weakness, reduced mobility, and resistance to passive movements of the lips, mandible, and tongue were evident without signs of atrophy or fasciculations. The jaw and gag reflexes were considered brisk. Emotional incontinence was quite evident throughout testing. Articulation was severely slow-labored and imprecise, as were oral alternate and sequential motion rates. Phonation was harsh with intermittant periods of strained-strangled quality and arrests of phonation; mono-loud and monopitch characteristics were also evident. Hypernasality and snorting were variably perceived.

Salient symptoms/signs	Test results	Impressions

This worksheet is to be used for recording relevant diagnostic observations. The blank illustration is to be used for identifying and sketching the suspected site of lesion(s). These steps should be completed prior to turning to the Impressions and illustrated site of lesion.

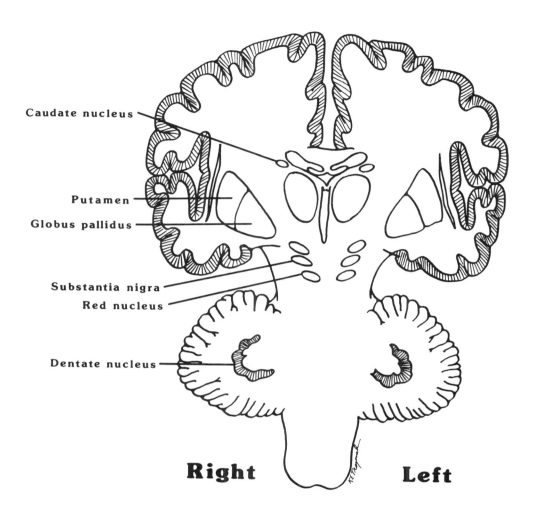

Caudate nucleus

Putamen

Globus pallidus

Substantia nigra

Red nucleus

Dentate nucleus

Right

Left

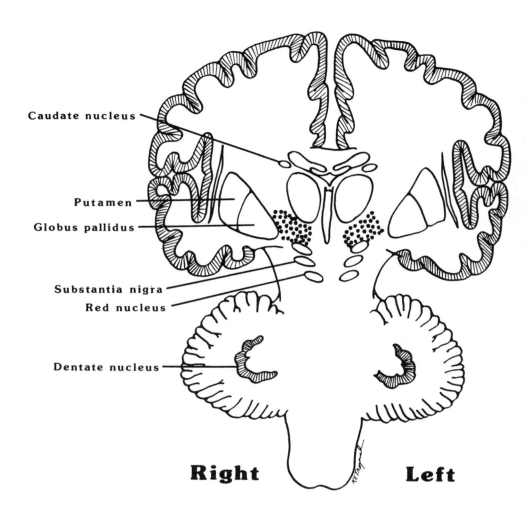

Caudate nucleus

Putamen

Globus pallidus

Substantia nigra

Red nucleus

Dentate nucleus

Right

Left

Impressions   Spastic dysarthria.

Discussion   Damage to the corticobulbar tracts bilaterally causes paresis, hypertonicity, and slowness of movement of involved musculature, and frequently emotional lability secondary to control disinhibition. This is often referred to as *pseudobulbar palsy* and the motor speech signs, *spastic dysarthria.* The prefix "pseudo" is used because some of the signs, including weakness, slowness, and limitations in range of movement may superficially resemble cranial nerve lower motor neuron impairments referred to as *bulbar palsy* and the motor speech signs, *flaccid dysarthria.*

In pseudobulbar palsy, multiple muscle groups are usually involved and the affected muscles are hypertonic and hyperreflexic. In bulbar palsy, muscles are hypotonic, hyporeflexive, and one or more muscles may be affected depending upon how many cranial nerves are damaged.

Articulatory impairment in each condition may be quite similar, while resonatory and phonatory features differ. In spastic dysarthria, velopharyngeal incompetence may be variable and the voice quality strained-strangled with intermittent periods of voice arrest. On vowel prolongation, the "wail" quality gives the examiner the impression of crying.

In flaccid dysarthria, depending upon the site and extent of involvement of the IXth and Xth cranial nerves, which subserve velopharyngeal and laryngeal function, resonation and phonation may be impaired. For example, unilateral involvement of the recurrent branch of the Xth nerve produces hoarseness and weak cough, while bilateral recurrent laryngeal nerve involvement may minimally impair voice but produce significant problems breathing. Continuous hypernasality, nasal emission and hoarseness-breathiness can be identified to varying degrees with IXth and Xth nerve involvement at the brainstem level. Because of the high risk for respiratory insufficiency and aspiration, patients with flaccid dysarthria sometimes require tracheostomy.

In this patient, drooling was thought to be a consequence of labial-lingual involvement with resultant difficulty propelling the bolus posteriorly. Nasal regurgitation was attributed to velopharyngeal involvement.

20-Year-Old Female with Closed Head Injury

History   The patient is a 20-year-old, right-handed, female who was entering her sophomore year in college in good health until she was found unconscious after a motor vehicle accident. An MRI of the head obtained on admission to the hospital revealed a shearing injury of the corpus callosum, focal contusion, hemorrhagic lesions involving the left thalamus, and contusions of the right cerebral cortex. She remained comatose for twenty days after the accident. After regaining consciousness, she was rated as Level V on the Ranchos Los Amigos Scale (confused, inappropriate, nonagitated). She was subsequently transferred to a rehabilitation facility near her home for comprehensive evaluation and treatment.

Examination   One month after the injury, the patient was alert, attentive, and well-oriented to day, month, and surroundings. Examination of the oral speech mechanism revealed normal functioning cranial nerves V (motor and sensory), VII, IX through XII. There were no pathologic reflexes. The structural integrity of the speech mechanism was sound for speech production. Articulation, phonation, resonation, respiration, and prosody were felt to be within normal limits; but the patient had a tendency to echo the examiner's questions or repeat her own utterances, frequently three to four times. Verbal expression was grammatically and semantically sound.

She had no difficulty following one-step through two-step complex instructions, nor did she have difficulty obtaining meaning from a multiple-word, complex paragraph. She could retain six digits forward and five backward and could repeat lengthy sentences. There was a question of a left visual field defect on double simultaneous stimulation testing; she had no difficulty reading or obtaining meaning from isolated words, simple to complex sentences, or a multiple-word, complex paragraph. She scored at the 82nd percentile on one neurocognitive measure. Neuropsychological testing revealed a verbal IQ of 79, a performance IQ of 63, and a full scale IQ of 72, suggesting low borderline cognitive skills.

Salient symptoms/signs	Test results	Impressions

This worksheet is to be used for recording relevant diagnostic observations. The blank illustration is to be used for identifying and sketching the suspected site of lesion(s). These steps should be completed prior to turning to the Impressions and illustrated site of lesion.

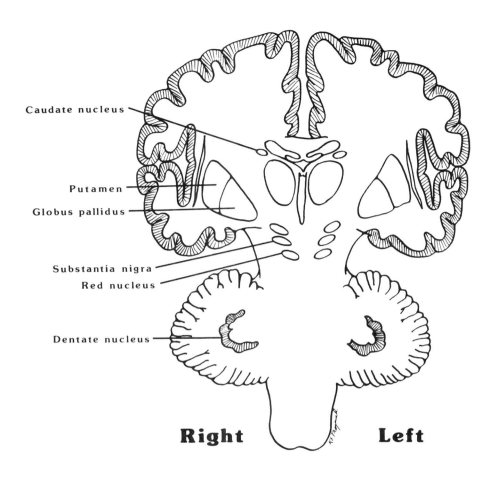

Caudate nucleus

Putamen

Globus pallidus

Substantia nigra
Red nucleus

Dentate nucleus

Right　　**Left**

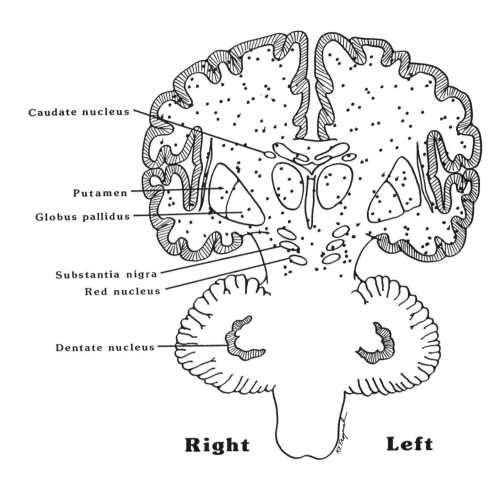

Caudate nucleus

Putamen

Globus pallidus

Substantia nigra

Red nucleus

Dentate nucleus

Right　　　**Left**

Impressions Confused language, with echolalia and palilalia one month following closed head injury; traumatic encephalopathy.

Discussion The clinical findings in this patient point to diffuse axonal injury with resultant diminution in communicative-cognitive function judged to be mild/moderate in degree. The presence of echolalia and palilalia (reiterative utterances characterized by word, phrase, or segment of phrase repetitions; forms of perseveration) are not uncommon in encephalopathy and may represent subcortical or diffuse bifrontal pathology. Palilalia seems to involve primarily words and larger units of language rather than sound or syllable repetitions, prolongations, hesitancy, and so on.

The patient was enrolled in an intensive inpatient and outpatient program of cognitive rehabilitation with significant gains made in all areas treated. At three months status post-closed head injury, performance was now between the 95th and 98th percentile on two cognitive measures. Neuropsychological reevaluation revealed a verbal IQ of 93, a performance IQ of 86, and a full scale IQ of 88, suggesting improvement in cognitive function—although based on her premorbid status, not normal for her. Pending further improvement in her cognitive status, she planned to return to college to complete her degree.

39-Year-Old Female with Frontal Headache and Unintelligible Speech

History While jogging, a slightly hypertensive left-handed 39-year-old house-wife experienced a sudden and severe frontal headache. She walked the rest of the way home, feeling very nauseated, dizzy, and faint. The throbbing in her head was not relieved with aspirin or ice pack. She attempted to phone her husband but was unable to speak clearly. She did, however, manage to convey that she was in pain. He rushed home and promptly took her to the hospital emergency room.

By then, her head movements were stiff and her speech was virtually unintelligible. However, she was able, by nodding her head, to answer simple yes or no questions. In the emergency room, her husband revealed his wife's hypertensiveness and that she had been placed on a low-salt diet and a moderate exercise program. Jogging had not been ruled out as harmful.

Examination The patient was mildly disoriented and confused during testing. She held her forehead to signal pain and discomfort. Her face was flushed and her pulse was full and slow with a blood pressure reading of 150/95. She had a temperature of 102°F. The right arm and leg were weak, with deep reflexes being brisk. A slight Babinski sign was noted on the right. Nuchal rigidity was evident. Volitional nonspeech movements of the lips, jaw, and tongue were mildly impaired. With the exception of mild right central facial weakness, there were no signs of involvement of the remaining speech musculature.

All cranial nerves appeared intact, as was the entire left side of the body. Spinal tap revealed bloody cerebrospinal fluid. Cerebral angiography disclosed an avascular zone in the inferolateral posterior left frontal lobe region. CT scan suggested subarachnoid blood.

In that the patient was in pain, speech-language testing was difficult. She could, however, correctly point to various body parts, following either spoken or written stimulus presentation. She was oriented to time, place, and person and was able to follow all commands used during examination.

Speech was plagued by slow, groping, and effortful articulatory patterns. Frequent false starts, hesitations, and repetitions of individual sounds and words were evident. Words made up of complex sound combinations evoked omissions and substitution errors that were highly inconsistent and variable. Transpositions of individual sounds within words or words within short phrases stimuli were common. When asked if she could write what she was feeling, the patient grasped the pen in her dominant left hand and wrote, "My head is killing me. I don't understand what is happening. Please help me."

Salient symptoms/signs	Test results	Impressions

This worksheet is to be used for recording relevant diagnostic observations. The blank illustration is to be used for identifying and sketching the suspected site of lesion(s). These steps should be completed prior to turning to the Impressions and illustrated site of lesion.

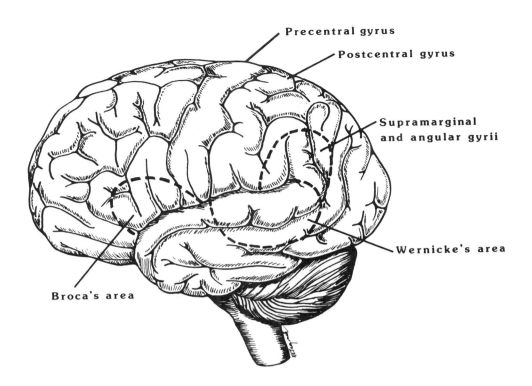

Precentral gyrus

Postcentral gyrus

Supramarginal
and angular gyrii

Wernicke's area

Broca's area

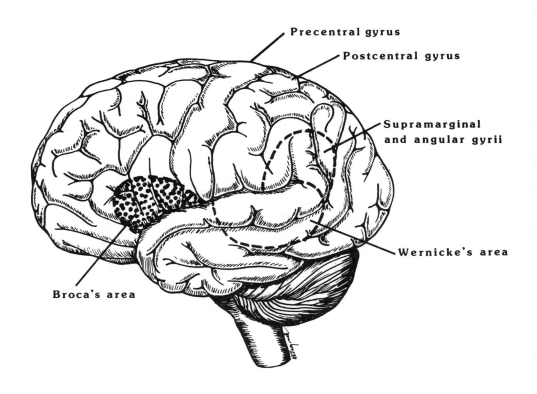

Precentral gyrus

Postcentral gyrus

Supramarginal
and angular gyrii

Wernicke's area

Broca's area

Impressions   Apraxia of speech secondary to an intracranial aneurysm.

Discussion   An intracranial aneurysm is characterized by a balloonlike dilatation of a cerebral blood vessel caused by a weakened vessel wall. These defects may be congenital in origin and may vary in size. Occasionally, an aneurysm may result from hypertension, arteriosclerosis, or emboli. More than half of all reported aneurysms are solitary and arise from the internal carotid or middle cerebral artery.

An aneurysm may be asymptomatic for many years, depending on its size and location. If it ruptures, the individual may experience an explosive headache resembling a migraine, nausea, stiff neck, or fever. Angiography and cerebrospinal fluid analyses are instrumental in illustrating cerebrovascular aneurysms and hemorrhages.

Our patient had a history of hypertension. Later it was learned that her father died of a ruptured intracranial aneurysm. A congenital asymptomatic defect in the walls of the middle cerebral artery was therefore suspected. The exertion and strain of jogging plus the hypertensiveness probably induced an increase in intravascular tension followed by rupture. The ascending frontal (sometimes called the candelabra) branch of the middle cerebral artery was felt to be the primary vessel of involvement. One month following insult, her clinical neurologic examination was judged normal; however, she continued to suffer from moderate expressive speech difficulties.

The diagnosis of apraxia of speech was reached, albeit with caution, at the time of the patient's admission to hospital. We felt that her articulatory characteristics and prosodic abnormalities lent support to the diagnosis. Moreover, her apparent preserved auditory, reading, and writing abilities prompted this impression.

As the patient recovered, the motor speech signs became clearer. She exhibited highly variable and inconsistent articulatory errors, most notably of the substitution and omission types. She groped and struggled to find the correct articulatory postures, especially on initial consonants of words. On a multisyllable word she exhibited variable transposition of sounds within the word. Sequential motor speech tasks, such as /mommy-baby-daddy/ were extremely difficult for her to repeat in the correct sequence.

She transposed sounds within and between words, and words within sentences, frequently rendering her speech ungrammatical. Her vocabulary was within normal limits and she spoke in full sentences, although they were characterized by false starts, articulation errors, and difficult words. Typical of apraxic speakers, she had long strings of intelligible, well-articulated speech.

Apraxia of speech is thought to be caused by damage to the inferolateral-posterior region of the frontal lobe, known as Broca's area, or the dominant supplemental motor cortex. Lesions in these areas may also produce a co-occuring oral apraxia marked by off-target movements of the oral musculature in attempts to complete a volitional act such as lip pursing, tongue wiggling, coughing, as was noted in this patient. The hemiparesis was consistent with left pyramidal tract involvement.

67-Year-Old Male with Pulmonary Disease, Headaches, Blurred Vision, Dizziness Syncope, and Speech Disturbance

History   The patient is a 67-year-old male admitted to the emergency room with a two- to three-week history of weight loss, intermittent headaches, and visual blurring. Four days prior to admission, he complained of dizziness; on the evening prior to admission he complained of severe headache and difficulty speaking. On the day of admission, he slumped forward without warning while eating his lunch. On regaining consciousness, within a couple of minutes, his communication was inappropriate. The patient's prior medical history is significant for chronic obstructive pulmonary disease (COPD) and a past history of cigarette smoking habit.

Examination   The patient was in no apparent distress on examination although somewhat uncooperative. Blood pressure, respiration, temperature, and fundoscopic examination were within normal limits. By startle examination, there was a question of a right visual field defect. Carotids were full without bruit. Ambulation was normal with no focal signs or pathological reflexes, although he was somewhat difficult to examine due to decreased cooperativeness.

Admitting CT scan both with and without contrast demonstrated an enhancing infiltrating lesion in the left temporal-parietal and anterior occipital lobe areas with surrounding edema. There was no appreciable midline shift or hydrocephalus. Chest x-ray was consistent with COPD.

The patient was notably anxious and frustrated concerning his communication deficit. His speech was essentially fluent, although periods of erroneous word selection, omissions, and agrammatism were apparent. He frequently strayed from the topic of conversation and seemed to respond without respect to the stimulus.

Examination of the motor speech mechanism proved unremarkable. The mouth was edentulous, but dentures were in place. None of the items used to assess oral or speech praxis was missed. Thirty percent of the items requiring understanding of right-left orientation and 80 percent of the items requiring knowledge of two-step complex commands were missed. Of the items requiring comprehension of prepositions and spatial relationships 10 percent were missed.

He was able to retain four digits forward but did not understand the task for testing digits backwards; 10 syllables and 9 words were retained. He recognized and comprehended isolated letters, while 30 percent of isolated words and 40 percent of simple-to-complex sentences were missed. He missed 40 percent of common objects and pictures of common objects to be named. Sixty percent of the items requiring mental calculation and 90 percent of the items requiring pencil-paper computation were missed. Twenty percent of the items requiring a copied response and 80 percent of the items requiring a written response to dictation were missed.

The patient was oriented to time, place, and person, although his communication problem interfered with performance and response utility.

Salient symptoms/signs	Test results	Impressions

This worksheet is to be used for recording relevant diagnostic observations. The blank illustration is to be used for identifying and sketching the suspected site of lesion(s). These steps should be completed prior to turning to the Impressions and illustrated site of lesion.

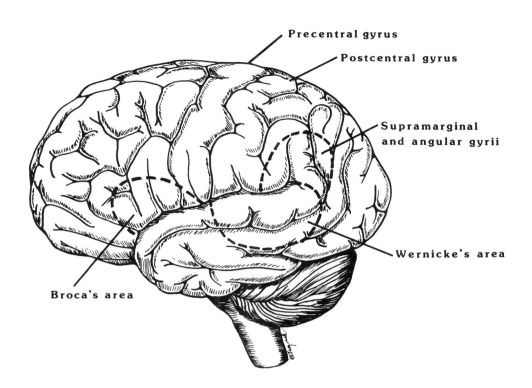

Precentral gyrus

Postcentral gyrus

Supramarginal
and angular gyrii

Wernicke's area

Broca's area

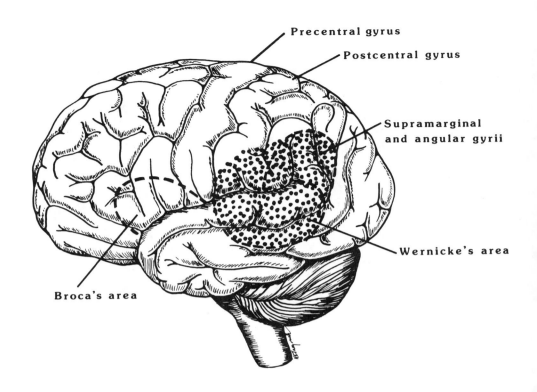

Precentral gyrus

Postcentral gyrus

Supramarginal
and angular gyrii

Wernicke's area

Broca's area

Impressions   Moderate aphasia due to neoplasm.

Discussion   The patient was discharged on dexamethasone (Decadron) and phenytoin sodium (Dilantin) for seizure precaution, and scheduled for readmission in six days for brain biopsy and possible excision of the lesion. Frozen section histology revealed primary CNS non-Hodgkins lymphoma. There was some improvement in language function postoperatively, although the patient remained dysphasic. An incomplete right homonymous hemianopsia was now apparent.

Radiation oncology was consulted and the patient was discharged and scheduled to be seen for full-course radiation therapy as well as outpatient speech therapy. His communicative status improved with radiation and speech therapy for approximately six months, at which time his health deteriorated, primarily because of his pulmonary disease. He eventually succumbed to bronchial pneumonia.

The language findings for this patient are fairly typical of aphasia in that the symptoms and signs crossed all language modalities. The absence of a motor speech deficit suggested that cortical and subcortical neuromotor control centers were spared from involvement by the neoplasm.

The efficacy of speech therapy is frequently challenged in cases of progressive or progressive degenerative illness, as in the case of this patient. To our knowledge, this question has not been addressed quantitatively but can be discussed empirically. It would seem that in conjunction with medical or medical-surgical management, speech therapy may provide maintaining as well as compensatory techniques and strategies for enhancement of communication, and therefore quality of life.

17-Year-Old Psychotic Male with Speech Disturbance

History A 17-year-old male was admitted to the psychiatric unit of a major hospital for observation and treatment following a six-month history of violent outbursts and an unprovoked attack on a neighbor. While in hospital, he remained agitated. In one instance, he attacked an orderly, requiring forceful restraint.

He was placed on fluphenazine enanthate (Prolixin) injection (1.25 mg 3 times daily) until symptoms were controlled, then oral maintenance therapy (Prolixin tablets, 2.5 mg 3 times daily) and gradually to 5 mg once daily. The regimen was maintained while the patient remained in hospital for three months and was continued for an additional five months following discharge. At the end of five months, he was seen for follow-up, at which time a change in speech was evident.

Examination Conversational speech was marked by moderately imprecise articulation, particularly at the ends of words, with distortion of both consonants and vowels. Oral diadochokinetic and sequential motion rates were slow and imprecise. Voice quality was harsh with variable increases in volume on isolated vowel prolongation. Speaking rate varied between fast and slow.

Variably slow-fast purse-string contraction of the lips, protrusion of the tongue, involuntary spasms of the periocular musculature (blepharospasm), and posturing of the mandible to the right was noted during speech examination. These movements could not be inhibited when called to the patient's attention. The remainder of the examination was unremarkable.

Salient symptoms/signs	Test results	Impressions

This worksheet is to be used for recording relevant diagnostic observations. The blank illustration is to be used for identifying and sketching the suspected site of lesion(s). These steps should be completed prior to turning to the Impressions and illustrated site of lesion.

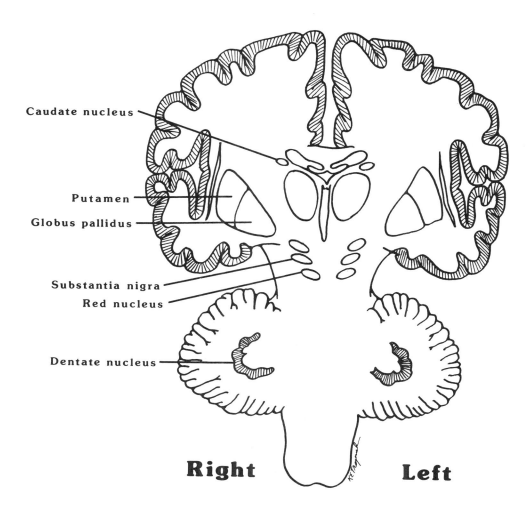

Caudate nucleus

Putamen

Globus pallidus

Substantia nigra
Red nucleus

Dentate nucleus

Right   **Left**

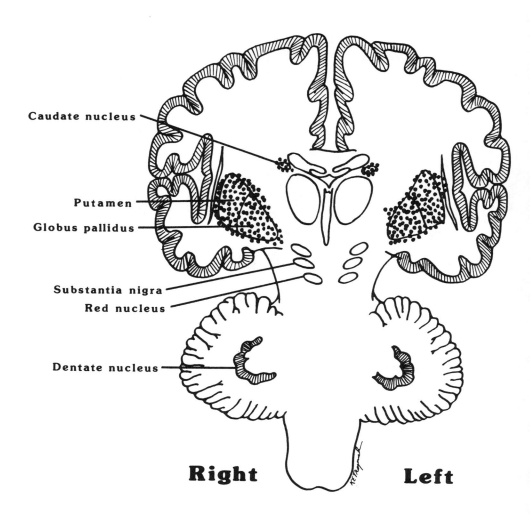

Caudate nucleus

Putamen

Globus pallidus

Substantia nigra

Red nucleus

Dentate nucleus

Right   **Left**

Impressions   Hyperkinetic slow dysarthria; tardive dyskinesia.

Discussion   Tardive dyskinesia is an iatrogenic (clinically or self-induced) disorder of movement associated with protracted use of phenothiazine, including Prolixin. The signs may occur during use of the drug or following withdrawal. Along with abnormal movements, signs such as cardiac arrhythmias, orthostatic hypotension, blurred vision, urinary retention, and sexual dysfunction may be noted.

In the hyperkinetic form, the movements may be choreatic and therefore quick and abrupt or dystonic and slow and sustained. A paucity of movement (hypokinesia) may be observed as well. The site of lesion is felt to be the striatum and globus pallidus within the basal ganglia. The actual pathogenesis of the dyskinesia, however, remains unknown.

In this patient, as is true with all patients with hyperkinetic dysarthria, the degree of speech impairment is directly related to the number and severity of involved muscles. For example, a focal dystonia involving the lower lip and face musculature may adversely affect bilabial productions and cause drooling, but preserve speech intelligibility. Conversely, a full-blown oro-buccal-lingual dyskinesia may significantly distort all speech sounds, thereby adversely affecting intelligibility as well as causing masticatory and deglutatory problems.

Treatment for tardive dyskinesia is essentially two-fold. First, the offending neuroleptic is discontinued. Second, reserpine, a dopaminergic blocker, may be used to help restore a dopamine balance. Since phenothiazines are prescribed for psychoses, patient monitoring for signs of affective as well as movement disorders is critical after such drugs have been discontinued.

68-Year-Old Female with Progressive Balance, Coordination, Hearing, Speech, and Swallowing Disturbances

History

Over the course of nine months, a previously healthy 68-year-old widow experienced progressive dizziness, unsteadiness, decreased hearing ability in the left ear, hoarseness, and swallowing and speech difficulties.

Examination

The patient denied a family history of similar symptoms. She remarked the symptoms began unexpectedly and had progressed slowly. When asked why she had waited so long before she sought help, she indicated that she thought her symptoms were normal and due to aging.

On physical examination the patient demonstrated the following: (1) moderate degree of weakness of the trapezius and sternocleidomastoid muscles, with an associated drooping of the left shoulder and difficulty rotating the head to the right; (2) a left vocal cord paralysis in the open position with associated atrophy, hoarseness, pitch breaks, reduced volume and stridor; (3) deviation of the tongue to the left upon protrusion, with an associated mild degree of weakness, atrophy and hypotonia on the left, and mild to moderate reduction in the range of motion, control, and speed of movements.

Articulation was imprecise, diadochokinetic rates were slow. Also noted: (4) deviation of the soft palate to the right at rest and during vowel prolongation, with associated mild hypernasal resonance; (5) anesthesia on the left side of the soft palate; (6) severe sensorineural hearing loss on the left side, with an absent caloric response on that side; and (7) difficulty with oral and pharyngeal transit during swallowing.

Laboratory tests included polytomography of the internal acoustic canals, arteriography, skull x-rays, and CT scan. The base of the skull x-rays and CT scan showed signs of a large mass occupying the area of the jugular foramen. It appeared that this mass had eroded a significant portion of the jugular and hypoglossal foramina. Arteriography indicated that this mass had extended into the cerebellopontine angle on the left; tomography revealed associated VIIIth nerve involvement.

Salient symptoms/signs	Test results	Impressions

This worksheet is to be used for recording relevant diagnostic observations. The blank illustration is to be used for identifying and sketching the suspected site of lesion(s). These steps should be completed prior to turning to the Impressions and illustrated site of lesion.

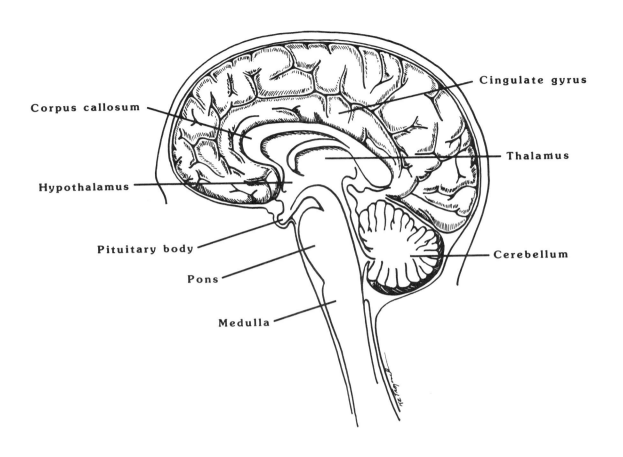

Corpus callosum

Cingulate gyrus

Hypothalamus

Thalamus

Pituitary body

Pons

Cerebellum

Medulla

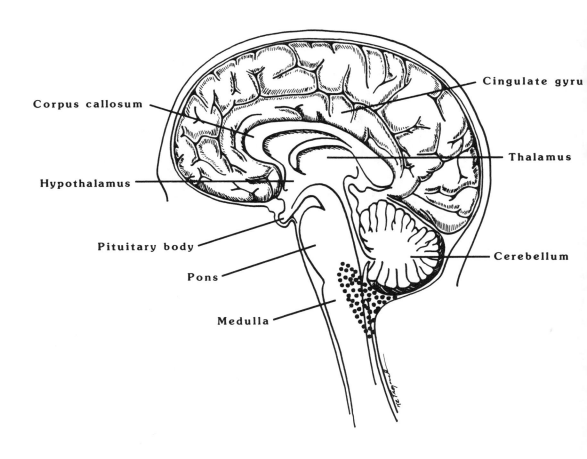

Corpus callosum

Cingulate gyru

Hypothalamus

Thalamus

Pituitary body

Pons

Cerebellum

Medulla

Impressions   Flaccid dysarthria secondary to neoplasm encompassing cranial nerves VII, IX, X, XI, and XII on the left.

Discussion   Surgery revealed a large tumor situated between the brainstem and base of skull on the left, associated with involvement of the cerebellopontine angle. The tumor was removed, but erosion of the jugular and hypoglossal foramina was irreversible, as were the paralytic effects the tumor had on the cranial nerves that exit the cranium through these openings.

Lesions of cranial nerves generally produce flaccid (bulbar) paralysis of the muscle(s) supplied. Atrophy, fasciculations, weakness, paralysis, and hypotonia and hyporeflexia of the involved musculature may occur in varying degrees, depending on the type, extent, and site of involvement. A lesion of a cranial nerve may occur anywhere from its nuclear origin in the brainstem throughout its course.

There are important differential diagnostic clues that help distinguish a lesion at the brainstem level (nuclear) from one involving the nerve after it has left the brainstem. Nuclear lesions of the cranial nerves, V, VII, IX, X, XI and XII, which innervate speech musculature, produce the classic signs of bulbar palsy or flaccid dysarthria. However, at the brainstem level, such lesions typically involve supranuclear structures as well, thereby causing co-occurring upper motor neuron (pseudo-bulbar palsy) signs.

Lesions that affect the brainstem, as in our patient, may extend into the posterior fossa through which course cranial nerves IX, X, XI and XII. At this level, flaccid paralysis of various speech musculature is not accompanied by co-occurring upper motor neuron signs, since the site of lesion does not affect the motor and sensory pathways of the central nervous system.

Our patient exhibited signs and symptoms of involvement of the VIIIth through XIIth cranial nerves on the left side. Acoustic nerve (VIII) findings included her hearing loss, dizziness, and unsteadiness. Glossopharyngeal nerve (IX) involvement was evident by the anesthetic palate on the left. High Vagal (X) nerve signs included open vocal cord paralysis with resultant dysphonia, and velar deviation with associated hypernasality: with unilateral weakness, the velum deviates, or is pulled, to the stronger side during vowel prolongation.

Spinal-accessory nerve (XI) dysfunction caused left shoulder droop and difficulty with head rotation to the right. Hypoglossal nerve (XII) involvement was evident by unilateral tongue weakness on the left: with unilateral weakness, the tongue deviates, or is pushed, by the stronger side to the weak side during protrusion.

Treatment included Teflon® injection of the paralyzed vocal cord to increase its bulk for approximation by the uninvolved cord, and speech therapy. Speech therapy emphasized compensatory articulation skills, better glottal resistance for initiating phonation, through pushing and posturing techniques, and improving velopharyngeal competence using a U-tube nasal air-flow device for visual biofeedback.

67-Year-Old Male with Progressive Memory and Language Disturbances

History A previously healthy 67-year-old farmer noted progressive difficulty remembering and thinking of correct words. He also experienced trouble calculating and keeping his checkbook in order. As he was becoming somewhat anxious and frustrated about this situation, he sought medical advice.

Examination With the exception of an incomplete right homonymous hemianopsia and obvious difficulty talking, the remainder of the neurologic examination was essentially within normal limits. CT scan suggested a lesion of increased density in the left posterior temporal-parietal and anterior occipital lobe areas. EEG revealed focal slowing in a broadly comparable area.

Assessment of language function revealed that 30 percent of the items requiring understanding of right-left orientation and 80 percent of the items requiring understanding of two-step complex commands were missed. The patient was unable to retain instruction beyond 10 syllables or 9 words. He recognized and comprehended 70 percent of isolated letters in words and 60 percent of simple-to-complex sentences visually. Forty percent of common objects and pictures could not be named accurately. Sixty percent of items requiring mental calculation and 90 percent of the items requiring pencil-paper computation were missed. Of the items requiring a written response to dictation, 80 percent were missed.

Conversation was marked by erroneous word selection, perseveration, and occasional jargon or neologistic distortion (new word creation). He frequently strayed from the thought and responses were rendered without respect to stimulus; he was noticeably anxious and aware of his deficits. Motor speech function was within normal limits.

Salient symptoms/signs	Test results	Impressions

This worksheet is to be used for recording relevant diagnostic observations. The blank illustration is to be used for identifying and sketching the suspected site of lesion(s). These steps should be completed prior to turning to the Impressions and illustrated site of lesion.

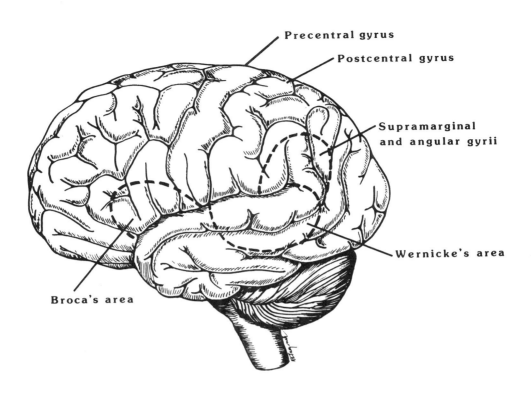

Precentral gyrus

Postcentral gyrus

Supramarginal
and angular gyrii

Wernicke's area

Broca's area

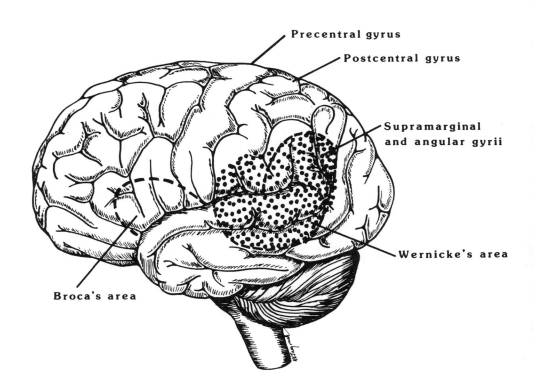

Impressions   Aphasia subsequent to a left hemisphere neoplasm.

Discussion   A lesion, in this case a Grade III glioma, involving the left midtemporal-parietal and anterior occipital lobe areas, resulted in aphasia crossing all language modalities. It is not uncommon for dysphasic signs to be categorized as unique language disorders—that is, dysnomic aphasia, auditory aphasia, and so forth. Because careful examination usually reveals that the aphasia crosses all language modalities, prefixes like "auditory," "dysnomic," etc. can be misleading.

A description of the specific findings as they exist as features of the disorder may prove less confusing diagnostically and more applicable therapeutically. Those rare syndromes—including alexia with and without agraphia, and pure word deafness—that selectively involve specific areas of language should not be confused with the multimodality language impairment of aphasia.

This patient's right homonymous hemianopsia points to a lesion beyond the optic chiasm involving the left optic nerve pathway, left occipital lobe, or optic radiations beyond the calcarine fissure on the left. His tumor was extirpated and he received focal radiation therapy. Unfortunately, he was left with aphasia that has responded slowly to speech therapy. At the time of this report, he continued to be followed by members of the neurosurgery, neurology, and speech pathology staff.

32-Year-Old Female with Transient Episodes of Dizziness, Incoordination, Neck Pain, and Speech Disturbance

History A 32-year-old housewife had a six-month history of transient dizziness, incoordination, indistinct speech, and neck pain. These conditions were being treated as psychosomatic. Over the course of the next three months, she experienced progressive and unrelenting chronic neck pain, jerking and weakness of the legs and arms, dizziness, difficulty walking, and slurring of speech, necessitating further medical advice.

Examination The patient was alert and cooperative throughout testing and her use of language was age-appropriate. She commented that, until the past months, that days and sometimes weeks might go by without any symptoms. Currently, however, she has become progressively more disabled.

Examination revealed: (1) wide-based and high steppage gait, particularly on the right, with associated circumduction of the right leg; (2) hypertonus and exaggerated muscle-stretch reflexes of the upper and lower limbs; (3) bilateral Babinski signs; (4) weakness of the arms and legs, without evidence of atrophy or fasciculations; (5) slow and irregular alternate motion rates of the upper and lower limbs; (6) reduced mobility of the soft palate, bilaterally, without signs of atrophy; (7) hyperactive gag reflex; (8) reduced range and mobility of the tongue without signs of atrophy or fasciculations; (9) mild-to-moderate increased resistance to passive tongue movements; (10) tongue weakness; (11) slow and dysrhythmic lingual and labial alternate motion rates; (12) articulatory imprecision; (13) prosodic insufficiency, characterized by outbursts of pitch and loudness changes particularly noticeable on vowel prolongation; and (14) harsh voice quality.

Laboratory tests showed an elevated level of gamma globulin. CT scan, skull x-ray, and cerebral angiography results were normal.

Salient symptoms/signs	Test results	Impressions

This worksheet is to be used for recording relevant diagnostic observations. The blank illustration is to be used for identifying and sketching the suspected site of lesion(s). These steps should be completed prior to turning to the Impressions and illustrated site of lesion.

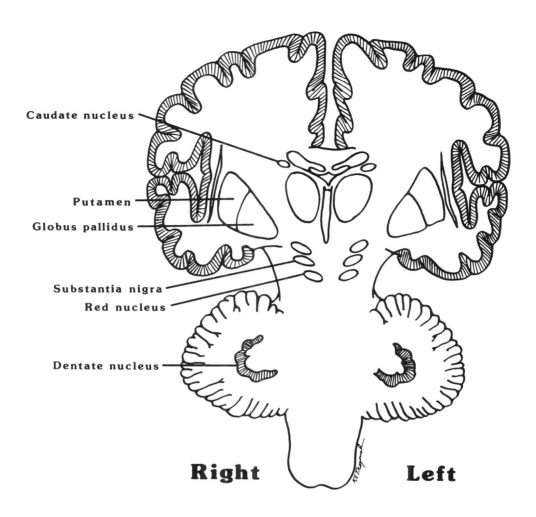

Caudate nucleus

Putamen

Globus pallidus

Substantia nigra

Red nucleus

Dentate nucleus

Right

Left

32-Year-Old Female with Transient Episodes of Dizziness, Incoordination, Neck Pain, and Speech Disturbance

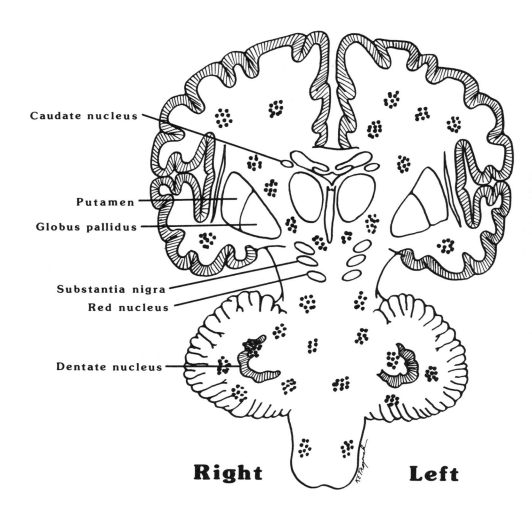

Caudate nucleus

Putamen

Globus pallidus

Substantia nigra
Red nucleus

Dentate nucleus

Right   **Left**

Impressions   Mixed spastic-ataxic dysarthria, caused by multiple sclerosis.

Discussion   Multiple sclerosis (MS) is a diffuse, slowly progressive disease due to demyelinization of axon sheaths of upper motor neurons. Onset is typically within the third or fourth decade of life. Following waxing and waning of symptoms in the early stages of the illness, exacerbations almost always occur, and become protracted with time. Although the etiology and pathogenesis of MS is still not clear, such factors as infections, lead poisoning, and dietary deficiency have been considered.

The pathologic effect of MS consists of multiple, well-defined areas of plaque formation (degeneration) in the white matter of the brain and spinal cord. The peripheral nervous system is usually uninvolved. The areas of degeneration vary in extent from microscopic size to more than 2 cm in diameter.

The degeneration of the myelin sheaths may vary from simple swellings to complete disappearance of the axons involved and subsequent scar formation. Such degeneration has a predilection for certain areas in the central nervous system. These include the: (1) optic nerves; (2) brainstem, and in particular the medial longitudinal fasciculus and corticobulbar tracts; (3) cerebellum; and (4) posterior columns and corticospinal tracts within the spinal cord.

The typical symptoms of MS include visual disturbances with associated pain in the eyes, tremor, ataxia, paresis, hypertonicity, weakness, dysarthria, and bladder incontinence. The diagnosis of MS relies on specific clinical considerations including: (1) neurological evidence of dysfunction in more than one site of the CNS; (2) a relapsing and remitting course of symptoms; (3) a slow or stepwise progression of symptoms over, at least, six months; and (4) an onset usually between the ages of 20 and 50 years.

Our patient had been initially diagnosed as having a psychosomatic reaction. This conclusion was probably based on the waxing and waning of characteristics of her symptoms. Unlike many patients with MS, she did not exhibit signs of visual impairment. The laboratory data provided necessary differential diagnostic information, since the presence of neoplasms or other disorders to which her symptoms may have been attributed had to be ruled out.

Elevated levels of gamma globulin are highly correlated with both MS and syphilis. Our patient had an abnormally high gamma globulin count. The advent of magnetic resonance imaging (MRI) has considerably enhanced the means available for diagnosing MS.

A high-steppage gait (foot drop gait) is one in which the foot is raised high and is suddenly lowered, thereby forcing the sole to strike the ground in a flapping fashion. In our patient, both this condition and the wide-based (ataxic) gait suggested cerebellar impairment. In terms of speech, the prosodic abnormalities and dysrhythmic oral alternate motion (diadochokinetic) rates also implicated the cerebellum.

Co-occurring with the cerebellar signs were the pathophysiologic effects of pyramidal system (corticobulbar and corticospinal tract) involvement. Specifically, these were manifested by: (1) exaggerated reflexes, (2) Babinski signs, and (3) limb and speech musculature hypertonicity, weakness, and paresis.

Because the course of MS is varied and unpredictable from one patient to another, our patient's progress is uncertain. However, the average survival after onset of symptoms is approximately 27 years.

69-Year-Old Male with a Ten-Day History of Difficulty Talking, Along with "Confusion"

History This 69-year-old, right-handed male who has a 50-year history of tobacco use and mild degenerative joint disease, was observed by his wife to have difficulty expressing himself and accurately completing business-related matters for ten days before being seen. She also felt that as of late he had been sleeping more. Approximately fifteen days before being seen, he had fallen while descending stairs, but did not sustain any recognizable injury or loss of consciousness. He had continued to drive to and from work without difficulty. There were no complaints of limb weakness, nausea, vomiting or change in bladder or bowel function. There had been no apparent seizure activity. At the time of examination, he was taking steroids for occasional arthritic pain.

Examination The patient was attentive, compliant, and well-kempt on examination and in no acute distress. With the exception of the communicative signs, there were no other findings on neurologic examination. Chest x-ray was normal. Neuroimaging studies were pending at the time of the speech pathology examination.

The patient was somewhat labile, and when asked to describe his difficulty with communication, he said: "I can't talk right." The structural integrity of the speech mechanism was sound for speech production. None of the items used to assess oral or speech praxis were in error, although the patient had a tendency to abort tasks prematurely saying: "I can't do that." Limb praxis was normal.

Expressive language was frequently agrammatical and characterized by omission of function words, such as and, or, the, etcetera. Erroneous or new words were frequently added to his utterances.

Eighty percent of the items requiring comprehension of single, one-step verbal commands were accurate, with only forty percent of the items requiring knowledge of right-left orientation accurate. He was unable to follow two-step, complex commands or obtain meaning from a multiple-word, complex paragraph. There was a question of an incomplete right visual field defect on both single and double simultaneous visual stimulation testing. Visual comprehension skills were very similar to those demonstrated during auditory comprehension testing; the majority of simple, one-step printed or written commands were accurate, although he was unable to obtain meaning from simple to complex sentences or a multiple-word, complex paragraph. None of the items requiring a verbal label for a common object or pictures thereof were accurate. From dictation, he was able to write his name and 40 percent of simple common words without error. He could not write phrases or sentences to dictation or write a story about an action picture shown to him. Forty percent of the items requiring mental or paper and pencil computation were accurate; he was unable to complete complex arithmetic forms. Perseveration was noted for both writing and computational tasks.

Salient symptoms/signs	Test results	Impressions

This worksheet is to be used for recording relevant diagnostic observations. The blank illustration is to be used for identifying and sketching the suspected site of lesion(s). These steps should be completed prior to turning to the Impressions and illustrated site of lesion.

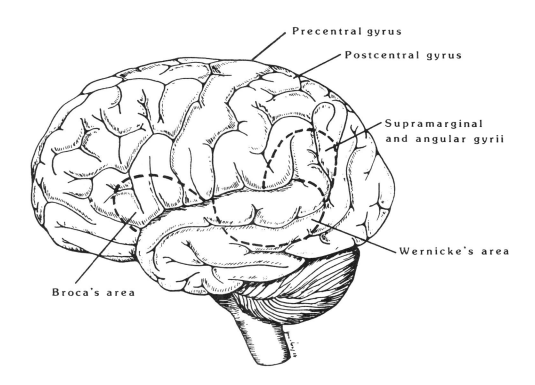

Precentral gyrus

Postcentral gyrus

Supramarginal
and angular gyrii

Wernicke's area

Broca's area

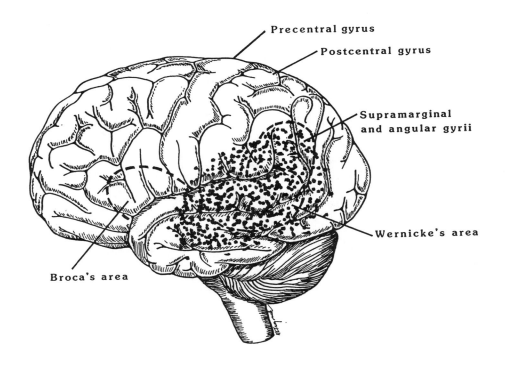

Precentral gyrus

Postcentral gyrus

Supramarginal
and angular gyrii

Wernicke's area

Broca's area

Impressions   Dysphasia, moderate/severe in degree secondary to a left cerebral hemispheric lesion; neoplastic process, brain tumor.

Discussion   The patient's history and progressive process of symptoms, point to a neoplastic process. Both CT and MRI imaging of the brain revealed an irregularly enhancing mass involving the midtemporal, parietal, and anterior occipital lobe areas of the left cerebral hemisphere. He was subsequently taken to surgery where, through craniotomy, a tumor was debulked and as much abnormal brain removed as possible. Pathology revealed glioblastoma multiforme, in this case rapidly aggressive.

After a brief period of healing and convalescence, the patient was seen for outpatient, full-course radiation therapy. Being at risk for seizures and brain edema, he was also started on anticonvulsive therapy and steroids.

Even though radiation therapy began soon after his surgery, at two months after removal of the tumor, his status declined rapidly and he was placed in a hospice for terminal care. Because of the rapidly progressive nature of the disease process, he was not seen for formal language therapy. In this patient's case, his "confusion" was most likely a manifestation of the dysphasia; the visual field signs suggested involvement of the occipital lobe and optic radiations of the left cerebral hemisphere.

77-Year-Old Male with Progressive Memory, Attention, Language, and Speech Disturbances

History The patient is a 77-year-old male who was referred for neurologic evaluation by his internist. His chief complaint was that over the past two years he has had problems with his "nerves" and has had difficulty sleeping. He is described by his daughter as being somewhat of a recluse, occasionally stumbles when turning around, stutters, and may "slur some words."

He was a known hypertensive, and had been taking a diuretic type of antihypertensive medication for a number of years. Recently family members had noticed some diminution in memory, concentration, and attending skills. At times, and disassociated with the situation, he has cried or laughed.

Examination Clinical examination revealed masklike facies with some cogwheeling noted in the nuchal musculature. He was well oriented to time, place, and person, although he did not know who the president was nor how many states were in the union. Glabellar, sucking, jaw-jerk and palmomental reflexes were positive. Cogwheeling rigidity was also noted at the wrists and elbows, bilaterally. Deep tendon reflexes were mildly brisk while knee jerks were moderately brisk, bilaterally. Sensory examination was within normal limits. Gait was marked by a rather stooped posture with short steps and loss of arm swing.

A CT scan could not be obtained on the day of clinical examination; therefore, this was rescheduled along with speech pathology examination because of the noted change in his communicative skills. However, one week prior to reexamination, the patient slipped at home and fractured his right femur, necessitating hospitalization.

On follow-up examination during hospitalization, periodic adventitious movements of the perioral musculature were noted to accompany the masked facies. Lip strength was mildly reduced. Bulbar reflexes were brisk. Articulation in context was variably imprecise and marked by inconsistent articulatory breakdown secondary to omission , distortion, and prolongation of individual sounds and occasional repetitions of entire phrases.

Oral diadochokinetic and sequential motion rates were accelerated and moderately irregular. Speaking rate was increased in segments, with short rushes of speech and inappropriate silent intervals. Phonatory function was marked by mildly reduced cough and hard glottal attack. The volume and pitch were reduced. A trace of variable hypernasality was noted.

Although the patient's language function was grammatically and semantically sound, his general fund of knowledge appeared reduced and tasks requiring abstract thought suggested concretism. Neuropsychological testing revealed reduced verbal and performance IQ, rendering a rather flat intelligence profile.

Throughout the examination the patient was attentive and cooperative; he denied depression, although he cried inappropriately and without respect to stimulus. EEG showed mild diffuse slowing. CT scan revealed enlargement of the left lateral ventricle and hypodensity in the right and left basal ganglia.

Worksheet

Salient symptoms/signs	Test results	Impressions

This worksheet is to be used for recording relevant diagnostic observations. The blank illustration is to be used for identifying and sketching the suspected site of lesion(s). These steps should be completed prior to turning to the Impressions and illustrated site of lesion.

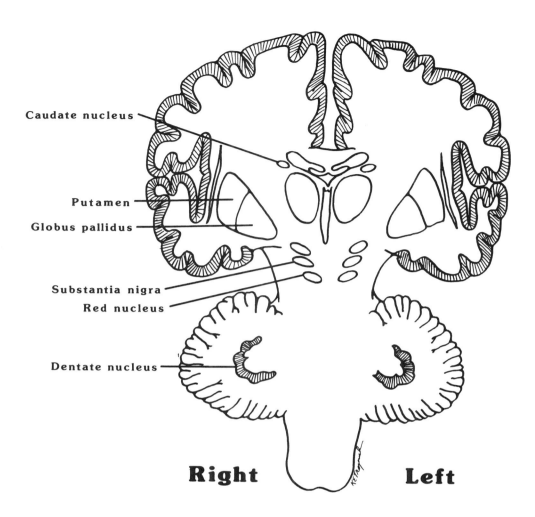

Caudate nucleus

Putamen

Globus pallidus

Substantia nigra

Red nucleus

Dentate nucleus

Right　　　**Left**

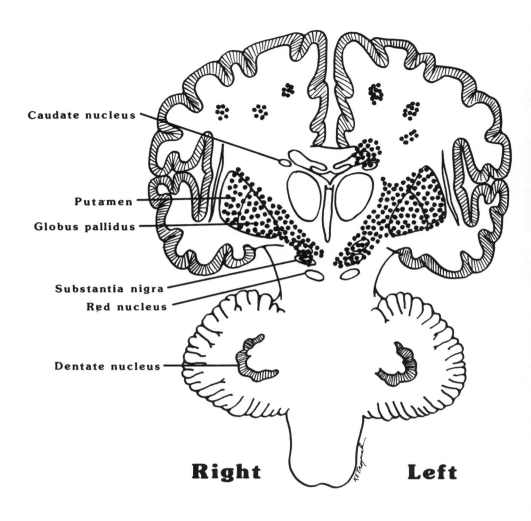

Caudate nucleus

Putamen

Globus pallidus

Substantia nigra

Red nucleus

Dentate nucleus

Right   **Left**

Impressions   Hypokinetic dysarthria and generalized intellectual impairment due to multiple infarction.

Discussion   In this case, the CT scan provided the differential diagnosis. The results revealed dilatation of the anterior portion of the left lateral ventricle and loss of brain tissue compatible with an old infarction. A number of low density areas in the anterior portion of the left and right basal ganglia and distal white matter were also noted.

Additionally, there was a small amount of blood (hematoma) in the posterior portion of the occipital horn of the right lateral ventricle. Repeat CT scan the following day revealed a decrease in the amount of blood in this area and reconfirmed the multiple sites of infarction.

The cause of this patient's vascular disease was most likely hypertensive. Dementia in late stages of idiopathic Parkinson's disease is not uncommon, however, and needs to be differentiated from other dementing illnesses, particularly dementia of the Alzheimer type and Creutzfeldt-Jakob disease, in that course may be more rapid and the mortality greater in the latter.

Although the behavioral diagnosis of dementia is usually based on memory and cognitive signs, this patient's speech was particularly impressive. The dysarthria was of the hypokinetic type, as seen in Parkinson's disease or parkinsonism, and the palilalic features (repetition of phrases and sentences) characteristic of diffuse/multifocal encephalopathy. The pseudobulbar lability was indicative of pyramidal tract involvement, while the other axial and appendicular skeletal signs were compatible with pyramidal and extrapyramidal involvement.

Unfortunately, patients with parkinsonian features secondary to vascular disease usually do not improve significantly with anticholinergic or dopaminergic drugs. Hypertensive medications may decrease the risk of subsequent infarctions.

73-Year-Old Male with History of Rheumatic Heart Disease Presents with Language Disturbance

History The patient is a 73-year-old male who, two days prior to admission, noted that he was repeatedly dropping things from his preferred right hand and had also decreased sensation involving the right hand to just below the elbow. One day prior to the examination, he rather consistently selected the wrong tools to work on his truck, and reversed numbers while writing a check. His local physician found normal right grip strength without decrease in sensation and felt the problem might be mechanical in origin. He referred the patient for orthopedic evaluation, which was normal. The orthopedist, however, felt that the patient may have experienced a mild stroke, and neurologic consultation was recommended.

Prior medical history was significant for rheumatic heart disease at age 40 with resultant heart murmur. He used alcohol moderately, and smoked one package of cigarettes per day for twenty years. A workup for endocarditis proved negative.

Examination Blood pressure was 170/90. There were no hypertensive changes. Fundi were normal. Bilateral carotid bruits, greater on the left than on the right, were evident; carotid pulse was good. Cranial nerves II through VII were clinically normal. Motor examination revealed mild weakness in the right biceps and comparable hypesthesia with decreased vibration sensation in the ankles, bilaterally. There was a slight decrease in fine motor control involving the right hand. Right pronator drift and poor handwriting skills were evident. There were no pathologic reflexes. The initial impression was transient ischemic attack (TIA).

Angiography revealed 50 percent stenosis of the left internal carotid artery with virtually no cross-circulation through the Circle of Willis. An endarterectomy was performed, but the postoperative course was complicated by what appeared to have been an ischemic event secondary to embolization. The patient was left with a dense right hemiparesis, comparable homonymous hemianopsia, and communicative difficulty.

CT scan revealed a large area of infarction involving the posterior-lateral margins of the frontal lobe and temporal-parietal lobes on the left. The patient was stabilized and transferred to the rehabilitation medicine unit for evaluation and therapy.

Speech pathology examination revealed marked right facial asymmetry with depression of the nasolabial fold on that side, but without compromise in the frontalis or superior margins of the right orbicularis oculi muscle. Cranial nerves V, IX, X, XI, and XII were clinically within normal limits. The right maxilla and mandible were hypesthetic to light touch.

The patient accurately followed simple one-step commands involving body parts and common objects. Simple linguistic formation, primarily isolated letters and words presented in the left visual field, were interpreted without difficulty. He was unable to calculate mentally or write with the right (preferred) upper extremity. Knowledge of time, place, and person, as well as assessment of memory were equivocal due to the pronounced language impairment. Attempts at speech were marked by considerable articulatory groping and off-target sound selection. Speech was intelligible primarily for simple monosyllabic words, such as "me," "I," and so on. Beyond this, errors consisted of sound and syllable transpositions, articulatory groping, and sound additions. A test of oral praxis revealed a 90 percent error.

In response to his inability to perform these tasks, the patient frequently became tearful or shook his head. In that speech output was significantly reduced, assessment of prosody was equivocal. Resonation, phonation, and respiration were felt to be adequate for ongoing speech.

Worksheet

Salient symptoms/signs	Test results	Impressions

This worksheet is to be used for recording relevant diagnostic observations. The blank illustration is to be used for identifying and sketching the suspected site of lesion(s). These steps should be completed prior to turning to the Impressions and illustrated site of lesion.

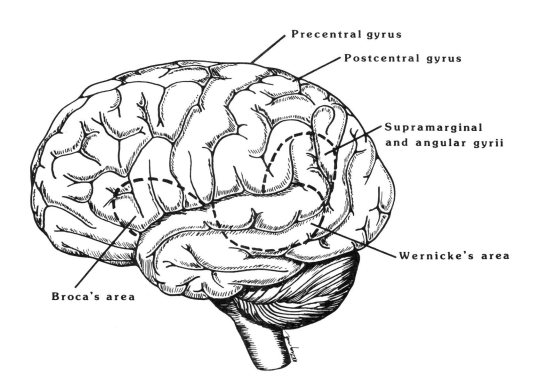

Precentral gyrus

Postcentral gyrus

Supramarginal
and angular gyrii

Wernicke's area

Broca's area

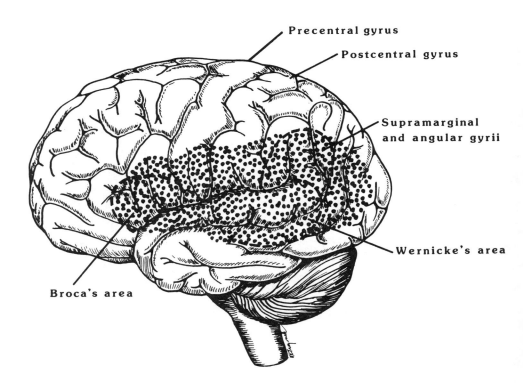

Precentral gyrus

Postcentral gyrus

Supramarginal
and angular gyrii

Wernicke's area

Broca's area

Impressions Speech/oral apraxia with comparable aphasia due to left hemisphere infarction.

Discussion Patients with a history of rheumatic heart disease are at high risk for vascular problems. It is conceivable that the endarterectomy caused, what appeared to be, an embolic stroke. The patient's verbal output was significantly reduced. His attempts at speech, along with his apparent recognition of the errors, even in the presence of a dense aphasia, are rather typical of a motor speech planning disorder—namely, apraxia of speech. Frequently, in severe involvement, it is quite difficult to differentiate between a motor planning and language-based deficit.

An index that frequently proves fruitful is to observe carefully the patient's response to errors. Frustration, frequent depression, or lability suggest that the patient is aware of the deficits.

The right side paresis and homonymous hemianopsia are compatible with the large left hemisphere lesion (middle cerebral artery distribution) that involved the pyramidal tract, and the post calcarine occipital lobe. The sensory impairment involving the right face is compatible with left parietal lobe involvement. Interestingly, central facial sensory impairments frequently are undetected because of co-occuring central facial paresis. What may be perceived as numbness by the patient may actually be weakness, or vice versa. On a supranuclear basis, the sensory pathways for the Trigeminal nerve (Vth) are primarily crossed, thereby explaining the contralateral hypesthesia.

The outlook for functional communicative recovery is generally poorer when both language and motor speech are involved, particularly to the degree that they are in this patient. However, patients who have a single embolic stroke seem to do better with therapy than those who experience a hemorrhagic or thrombotic infarct. At the time of this report, the patient's motor speech and language difficulties remained moderate in degree.

56-Year-Old Female with Progressive Voice Disturbance

History   A 56-year-old female music instructor sought laryngologic examination because of progressive hoarseness-breathiness and limited range of pitch beginning five weeks earlier. Following examination, the patient was assured that the voice signs were secondary to moderate bilateral vocal cord nodules and that with voice therapy or surgical vocal cord stripping she could expect a return of normal voice.

A period of voice therapy proved equivocal in alleviating the voice signs or size of the nodules; she therefore elected to undergo nodulectomy. Prior to surgery a baseline audiotape recording of the patient's voice was made, which revealed rhythmic changes in amplitude (intensity) averaging 5 Hz on prolongation of the vowel /a/, and mildly irregular oral diadochokinetic and sequential motion rates.

Examination   Following surgery the patient was seen for speech pathology consultations that revealed a decrease in hoarseness and breathiness, but maintenance of decreased pitch, regular changes in voice amplitude on vowel prolongation, and irregular oral diadochokinetic and sequential motion rates. The remainder of the motor speech examination was unremarkable. There were no signs of psychosocial discord nor was she depressed. Neurologic examination was significant only for mild right upper extremity rigidity.

Worksheet

Salient symptoms/signs	Test results	Impressions

This worksheet is to be used for recording relevant diagnostic observations. The blank illustration is to be used for identifying and sketching the suspected site of lesion(s). These steps should be completed prior to turning to the Impressions and illustrated site of lesion.

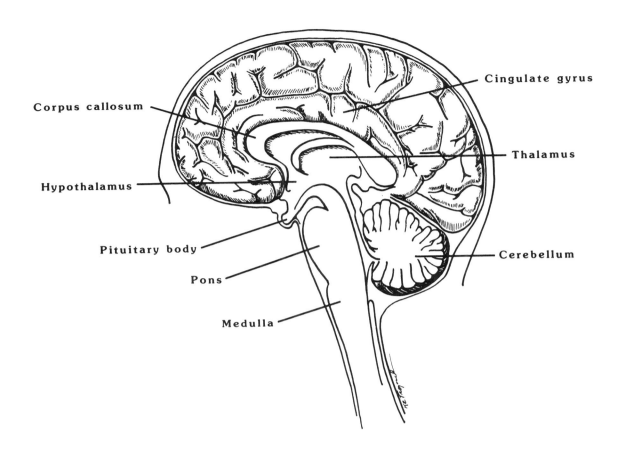

Corpus callosum

Hypothalamus

Pituitary body

Pons

Medulla

Cingulate gyrus

Thalamus

Cerebellum

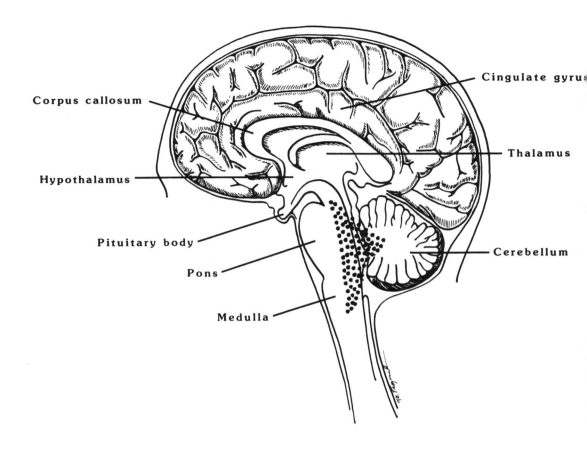

Corpus callosum

Hypothalamus

Pituitary body

Pons

Medulla

Cingulate gyrus

Thalamus

Cerebellum

Impressions   Hyperkinetic dysarthria; essential (voice) tremor.

Discussion   In this case, a mechanical defect masked subtle signs of neurologic disease. Essential tremor is a slowly progressive, nonfatal disease of unknown etiology that may result from lesions in different areas of the extrapyramidal system.

Some authors have ascribed the dentato-rubro-olivary tract as the primary site of lesion. The terms *benign* and *heredofamilial* are adjectives also used to describe the essential tremor syndrome. Initial signs may occur unilaterally in one limb, or, as in this case, the larynx. The term "benign" may be misleading in that in severe forms the disorder can prove significantly debilitating.

In severe forms of essential voice tremor, ongoing speech may be hindered by periodic complete adductory phonatory arrests, giving the voice a choking, strangled quality. The term adductor spasmodic dysphonia of essential (voice) tremor is used to differentiate the voice disorder from other voice disorders as well as from other forms of spasmodic dysphonia including focal laryngeal dystonia. Beta blocking agents including propranolol (Inderal) or ethanol may be helpful in alleviating tremor of the limbs, while methazolamide (Neptazane) may help the voice. Periodic botulinum toxin injections into the thyroarytenoid musculature is the standard of care for reducing adductor laryngospasms. Generally, for patients whose laryngospasm is related to tremor or who have focal laryngeal dystonia, the injections need to be repeated every 3 to 6 months.

54-Year-Old Male on Antidepressant Medication with Memory, Attentiveness, and Language Disturbances

History   The patient is a 54-year-old male who was referred to psychiatry for an evaluation of disturbed sleep, poor appetite, sexual dysfunction, constipation, profound fatigue, and difficulty concentrating on his work.

Initial psychiatric evaluation revealed depression thought to be associated with job stress. He was placed on a trial of antidepressants. Follow-up examination suggested improvement in depression; he was scheduled for reevaluation in two weeks. Within eight days, however, the patient complained of difficulty with memory and concentration on the job. He was admitted to the hospital for further evaluation.

Examination   The patient showed psychomotor retardation, depressed affect, and marked difficulty thinking of words, with resultant slowness of speech. General fund of knowledge appeared reduced.

Speech pathology examination revealed normal speech. Contextually, utterances were semantically and structurally sound, although hesitancies in context gave the appearance of a word-finding deficit. His comprehension and retention of multiple, progressively complex bits of information was age-appropriate. Comparable performance was also achieved on a word fluency measure. He did, however, have difficulty recalling instructions on a test of abstract thought. The latency of response was frequently up to 15 seconds per item.

Twenty percent of the items on a test of similarity were missed while 60 percent of the items requiring correction of erroneous and ambiguous sentences were missed. The patient was well oriented to time, place, and person, while 50 percent of the items used to assess long-term memory were missed. He did not know the president of the United States, or who discovered America, or the number of states in the republic. Affectively, he appeared depressed.

Neuropsychological testing revealed a verbal IQ in the dull-normal range with nonverbal IQ falling below this. His overall fund of knowledge was reduced. Further testing showed depression and anxiety embedded with an underlying obsessive personality.

Physical and neurologic examinations were well within normal limits. CT of the head and EEG were normal. It was felt that the original antidepressant regimen may have caused the patient to become hypotensive, thereby exacerbating some of his depressive symptoms. A different medication was prescribed and he was discharged to be followed as an outpatient by psychiatry.

On return examination to psychiatry, he demonstrated considerable difficulty recalling the names of his family or his place of employment. During conversation he would at times omit the first half of sentences making his communication rather tangential. Repeat neurologic examination as well as CT and EEG proved unchanged.

At this point, the patient's employment as a comptroller was in question, in that he was having considerable difficulty remembering the nature of his job and interacting with colleagues. He sought a second opinion from a nearby medical facility. The findings following evaluation there were essentially the same as those of the referring institution. He returned with his spouse for discussion of the probable diagnosis.

	Salient symptoms/signs	Test results	Impressions
Worksheet			

This worksheet is to be used for recording relevant diagnostic observations. The blank illustration is to be used for identifying and sketching the suspected site of lesion(s). These steps should be completed prior to turning to the Impressions and illustrated site of lesion.

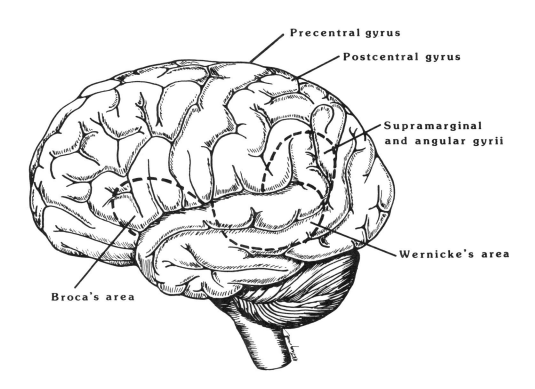

Precentral gyrus

Postcentral gyrus

Supramarginal
and angular gyrii

Wernicke's area

Broca's area

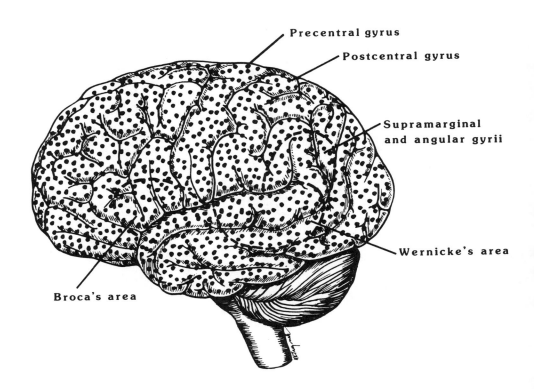

Precentral gyrus

Postcentral gyrus

Supramarginal
and angular gyrii

Wernicke's area

Broca's area

Impressions   Generalized intellectual impairment or dementia of the Alzheimer type, exacerbated by depression.

Discussion   Like many disorders of communication, personality, and affect, the diagnosis of dementia—including that of the Alzheimer type—is based on behavior. Specifically, the dementia is characterized by a decline in memory and other cognitive functions, although the former is frequently the chief presenting complaint.

Diagnosis of dementia of the Alzheimer type is one of exclusion; that is, other treatable illnesses must be ruled out as carefully as possible prior to rendering this diagnosis. The symptoms must not be confused with delirium or a change in consciousness; nor in the initial early stages can the diagnosis be made on the basis of focal cognitive or communicative deficits, such as dysphasia.

Although memory loss is a frequent early complaint of the disease, patients with Alzheimer's disease may only rarely complain of decrease in memory. In that memory loss may be a component of depression (which may be medically manageable), the patient complaining of this symptom should be followed carefully and receive psychiatric evaluation.

Along with psychiatric illness and focal neurological deficits, dementia of the Alzheimer type must be differentiated from other dementing illnesses, including normal pressure hydrocephalus, Creutzfeldt-Jakob disease, and schizophrenia.

With Alzheimer's disease, forgetfulness, confusion, and dementia are the primary cognitive behavioral symptoms. Other symptoms include: (1) a sense that "something is wrong" and increasing dependence on family members; (2) agitation and personality changes; and (3) withdrawal characterized by diminished levels of consciousness, incontinence, difficulty eating, inability to attain normal muscle tone, and progressive inanition (starvation) leading to death. It should be noted that distinguishable neurologic signs are frequently absent until only the advanced stages of the disease.

It is imperative that the patient suspected of having Alzheimer's disease be subjected to complete neuropsychological and laboratory study as well as routine neurologic and medical examination. Speech pathology examination may help elucidate language and, at a later stage, speech signs that may be embedded within the diffuse process.

At autopsy the brain of a patient with Alzheimer's disease rather consistently reveals neurofibrillary tangles and senile plaques. However, 20 percent or more of cases diagnosed clinically as having dementia of the Alzheimer type will at autopsy be found to have some other dementing illness. Further, tangles and plaques are not uncommon in the "normal" aged brain as well.

CT scan is useful for ruling out subdural hematomas, multi-infarct dementia, normal pressure hydrocephalus and brain tumors. Although not used universally as of yet, positron emission tomography (PET) and magnetic resonance imaging (MRI) may be potentially useful for differentiating dementia of the Alzheimer's type from other dementing illnesses.

Treatment of Alzheimer's disease remains just as elusive as its etiology. Medically, neuroleptic drugs have been used to reduce agitation and sleeplessness; tardive dyskinesias are not uncommon sequelae. Lecithin and oral physostigmine have been tried, with suggested improvement in memory. Recently intraventricular bethanechol has been used in a limited number of patients with reported improvement in the dementing signs.

While the medical community strives for adequate diagnostic and treatment measures for this severely debilitating disease, family and support groups such as the Alzheimer's Disease and Related Disorders Association remain in the forefront in the care of patients stricken with this illness.

67-Year-Old Female with History of Stroke and Heart Disease Presents with Acute Gait and Speech Disturbances

History
The patient is a 67-year-old female whose medical history is significant for a right hemisphere stroke and a long history of mitral valve stenosis. Since her stroke, which occurred approximately 15 years prior to this admission, the patient had done well. She lived alone and was able to cook and care for herself in spite of a partial left hemiparesis.

On day of admission, she was beginning to make breakfast when she became quite pale and, according to her grandson, who was staying with her, looked "very dizzy." Shortly after this, her speech became slurred and she had a difficult time walking. On transportation to hospital, the grandson noted that her breathing was irregular and that it was hard to get her to respond.

Examination
The patient presented to the emergency ward in a somewhat somnolent state, complaining of being tired. She was able to follow short directions and did not complain of dysphagia or, at this time, shortness of breath. She was well oriented. She was hyperreflexic on the left, but had normal reflexes on the right. Sensory and cerebellar examinations were within normal limits.

Chest x-ray showed cardiomyopathy and moderate pulmonary edema. Electrocardiogram revealed atrial fibrillation as well as left ventricuiar hypertrophy. Head CT scan revealed an old basal ganglion infarct on the right without further focal findings. The patient was transferred to the floor where she did well for the next 24 hours. On awakening at the beginning of the third day, she complained of mild right-sided weakness involving the arm and leg. Neurologic examination confirmed this. There were no sensory or cerebellar findings. The patient did well for the next 48 hours and was transferred to the rehabilitation medicine unit.

Examination revealed head and bilateral limb tremors at rest, at approximately 4 to 6 Hz. The neck appeared rigid and dorsiflexed. Her face lacked expression and appeared masked. On abduction of the lips, a residual right central facial paresis was evident. Lip seal and strength were mildly reduced with reinforcement. The mandible depressed to the midline without compromise in strength. The soft palate was symmetrical at rest and during phonation. The gag reflex was considered brisk. Tongue protrusion was to the midline, but moderately to severely reduced in strength; lateralization was comparably reduced.

Oral diadochokinetic and sequential motion rates were mildly slow and irregular, and rendered at a decreased amplitude. Variable and mild articulatory breakdown occurred secondary to sound distortion and decreased oral activity. Articulatory intelligibility was not significantly affected, although sounds were periodically distorted.

Phonation was marked by continuous severe breathiness and reduced loudness. Cough was considered mildly reduced. On prolongation of the vowel /a/ it appeared that voice quality was going to lapse into tremor, particularly at the termination of a sustained vowel. Laryngologic examination suggested normal cord abduction, but incomplete adduction. The cords appeared mildly bowed.

Respiration for speech was considered severely reduced with the length of the sustained /a/ less than 1 second. Speaking rate was considered decreased and reduced to phrases. In that utterances were brief, resonation was somewhat difficult to assess. At times it appeared that it lapsed into hypernasality with nasal emission.

Assessment of language function did not suggest a focal deficit. The patient was well oriented and missed none of the items used to assess long-term memory. She was periodically emotionally labile, both in terms of laughing and crying.

Worksheet

Salient symptoms/signs	Test results	Impressions

This worksheet is to be used for recording relevant diagnostic observations. The blank illustration is to be used for identifying and sketching the suspected site of lesion(s). These steps should be completed prior to turning to the Impressions and illustrated site of lesion.

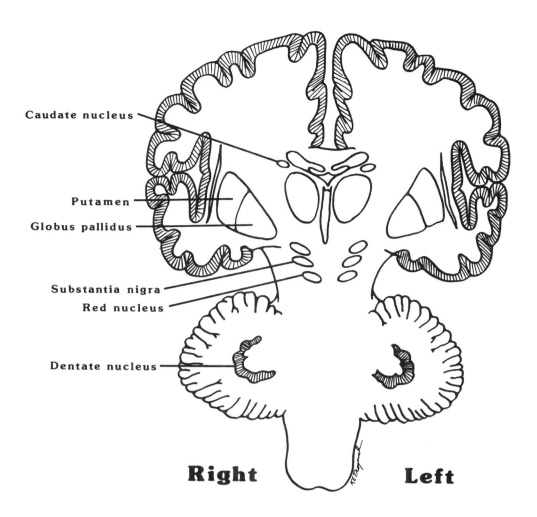

Caudate nucleus

Putamen

Globus pallidus

Substantia nigra

Red nucleus

Dentate nucleus

Right　　**Left**

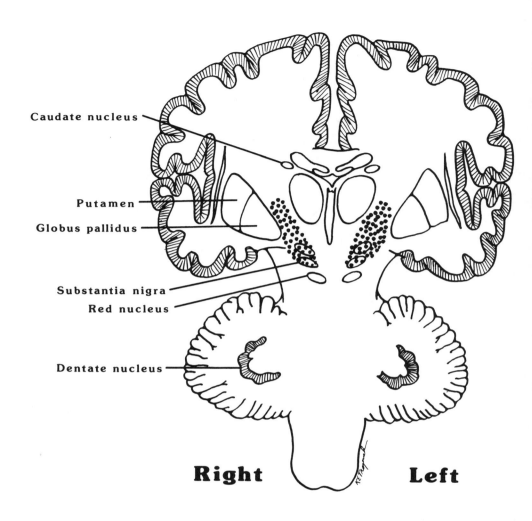

Caudate nucleus

Putamen

Globus pallidus

Substantia nigra
Red nucleus

Dentate nucleus

Right **Left**

Impressions   Mixed dysarthria of the hypokinetic and spastic types.

Discussion   The etiology of this patient's neurologic deficit appeared to be cardiovascular in origin, possibly related to an embolic event. Slow movement, paresis, and brisk reflexes are but a few clues suggestive of pyramidal system involvement, while masklike facies, tremor and rigidity are often indicative of basal ganglia disturbance. Likewise the slowed diadochokinetic and speaking rates and a question of hypernasality and nasal emission suggested spastic dysarthria, while the decreased range of diadochokinetic movements, decreased loudness, a question of voice tremor, and shortened utterances suggested hypokinetic dysarthria.

The articulatory imprecision was felt to reflect both dysarthrias. Patients who have vascular lacunar type parkinsonian features do not seem to benefit significantly from medical or speech therapy; their symptoms and signs are rather resistant to treatment. Fortunately for this patient, the mixed dysarthrias did not significantly interfere with speech intelligibility.

At time of discharge, the patient had regained only partial function of the right upper extremity while the left hemiplegia persisted and remained unchanged from admission. She was not able to walk independently, and she was fitted with a brace on the left ankle. She was placed on a medical regimen that included warfarin to prevent further strokes.

41-Year-Old Female with Progressive Shaking of the Limbs and Speech Disturbance

History A previously healthy 41-year-old woman scheduled an appointment because she developed progressive nonresolving shaking of the upper limbs and difficulty speaking during the course of 10 months.

Examination There was no familial history of a movement disorder. The onset of the symptoms was not precipitated by illness or accident. She was not taking prescribed medications, and used alcohol infrequently.

A moderate rest tremor of both upper limbs was observed that tended to dissipate with intention. Mild to moderate weakness and hypertonicity were evident in the upper limbs with associated cog-wheel rigidity and slow and reduced range of movement. Alternate motion rates of the fingers and hands were reduced in range and varied from rapid-fire and imprecise to slow and imprecise.

Gait was slow and marked by small steps. A mild horizontal rest tremor of the head was noted. The head and mandible showed moderate resistance to passive movements while volitional movements were moderately reduced in range, speed, and precision. Cranial nerve functions appeared normal, although she smiled infrequently.

Her language was age-appropriate. Her speech, however, was characterized by variable short rushes, inappropriate pauses between syllables and words, imprecise and variably slow-fast oral alternate and sequential motion rates, prolongations of vowels, and harsh, monoloud and monopitched phonation. Contextual speech was monotonous, lacked stress, and was periodically marked by consonant distortions. Thyroid function was normal. There was a question of increased density in the upper brainstem on CT scan.

Salient symptoms/signs	Test results	Impressions

This worksheet is to be used for recording relevant diagnostic observations. The blank illustration is to be used for identifying and sketching the suspected site of lesion(s). These steps should be completed prior to turning to the Impressions and illustrated site of lesion.

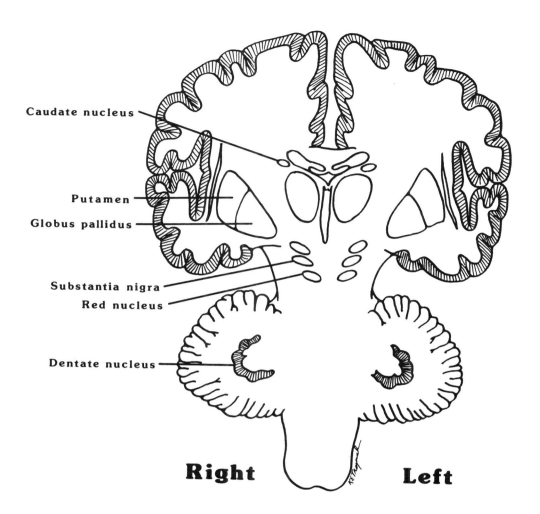

Caudate nucleus

Putamen

Globus pallidus

Substantia nigra
Red nucleus

Dentate nucleus

Right　　　　**Left**

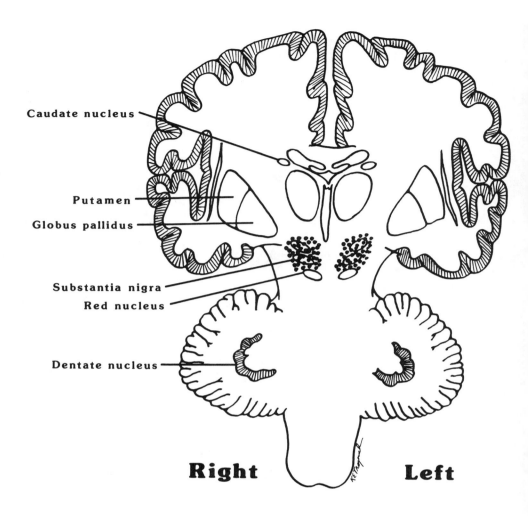

Caudate nucleus

Putamen

Globus pallidus

Substantia nigra
Red nucleus

Dentate nucleus

Right   **Left**

Impressions   Hypokinetic dysarthria associated with parkinsonism.

Discussion   Idiopathic Parkinson's disease is a slowly degenerative condition of middle age generally characterized by masklike expression and stiff facial movements, pill-rolling tremor of the fingers and wrists, hypokinesis and hypertonicity, cogwheel rigidity of the limbs, flexed truncal posture with associated slow-shuffling gait, and hypokinetic dysarthria.

Symptomatic parkinsonism, on the other hand, is the term used to describe Parkinsonianlike symptoms and signs that occur in the absence of the typical protracted history. In both conditions signs are associated with involvement of dopamine-rich cells of the striatum, substantia nigra, or both. The etiology of idiopathic Parkinson's disease is unknown; a slow virus has been postulated. Vascular, traumatic, metabolic, neoplastic, and toxic disturbances also have been implicated in parkinsonism.

In our case, a neoplasm in the region of the substantia nigra precipitated the progression of symptoms and signs observed. It may be hypothesized that as the area of the upper brainstem became increasingly compressed by the neoplasm, dopamine formation and function were suppressed. Parkinsonian hypertonia and hypokinesia caused by an imbalanced dopaminergic system consequently developed.

Cogwheel rigidity (as "cogs in a wheel") is characterized by a series of interrupting jerks of the arm or wrist as it is being passively flexed, extended, or rotated. Persistent abnormal stretch reflexes, possibly due to hyperfunctioning of the gamma system, is thought to underly these phenomena.

The dysarthria of idiopathic Parkinson's disease and symptomatic parkinsonism appears similar. Articulatory movements are variably slow-fast, reduced in range, and imprecise. Laryngeal and supralaryngeal vocal tract adjustments are similarly impaired, resulting in a harsh, monotonous voice pattern. The prosodic and contextual speech abnormalities reflect interactions among motor speech subsystems, including articulation and phonation. Patients with symptomatic parkinsonism seem to benefit less from dopaminergic replacement than do those with the idiopathic form of the disease.

73-Year-Old Female with Inability to Speak

History This 73-year-old, right-handed female was in excellent health until being seen in the emergency room with an acute inability to speak early that morning. She was accompanied by a friend who reported that one week previously the patient had complained of an intermittent headache. She had no headache on admission, however. The patient's prior medical history was noncontributory; there was no history of diabetes mellitus, hypertension, vascular disease, or stroke. She had been a widow for a number of years, had been living alone, and remained active.

Examination In the emergency room, the patient responded by gesturing yes/no with either her head or hand. She could not speak. Mild weakness of the lower two thirds of the face on the right and tongue deviation to that side on protrusion were evident. The patient drooled. Cranial nerve V (both motor and sensory) and VII (on the left) were functioning, although assessment of IX through XII proved equivocal, secondary to the communication impairment. The pharyngeal reflex was sluggish but elicited. Equilateral palmomental reflexes were elicited. Mild right upper and lower extremity paresis was evident. A Babinski sign was elicited on the right. EKG showed sinus tachycardia. Chest x-ray and heart size were normal. Neuroimaging studies were pending at the time of examination.

The patient was attentive and compliant although somewhat lethargic on examination. Because of the communication deficit, she could not elaborate on the history.

The patient made gross attempts at speech but could only approximate the target. For example, on assessment of oral diadochokinesis, she could approximate her lips but could not produce a neutral vowel afterward. She could not initiate voicing on request but frequently cleared her throat nonvolitionally. In summary, then, there were no instances of intelligible speech. None of the items used to assess oral praxis was accurate. Ninety percent of the items used to assess limb praxis were accurate with both upper extremities, although somewhat slower on the right side, secondary to paresis.

Using head or arm gestures, and eye gaze for response, assessment of auditory comprehension showed no deficits in her ability to follow simple, one-step through complex, two-step instructions or obtain meaning from a multiple-word, complex paragraph. For visual comprehension, none of the items requiring recognition or comprehension of isolated letters through simple to complex words and sentences was missed. Moreover, she had no difficulty obtaining meaning from a multiple-word, complex paragraph. Although there was no evidence of a visual field defect, gaze preference was to the left. Orthographic skills were affected by paresis of the right upper extremity. However, she was able to write her name, short words, and phrases legibly as well as the answers to simple arithmetic problems. The items requiring mental computation were accurate.

Salient symptoms/signs	Test results	Impressions

This worksheet is to be used for recording relevant diagnostic observations. The blank illustration is to be used for identifying and sketching the suspected site of lesion(s). These steps should be completed prior to turning to the Impressions and illustrated site of lesion.

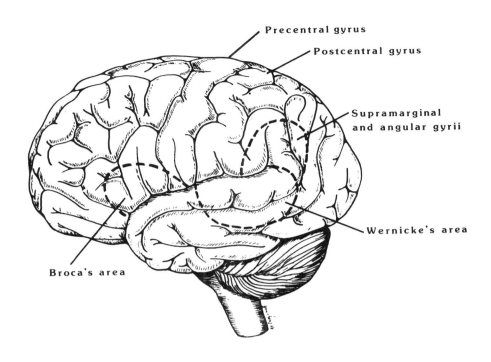

Precentral gyrus

Postcentral gyrus

Supramarginal
and angular gyrii

Wernicke's area

Broca's area

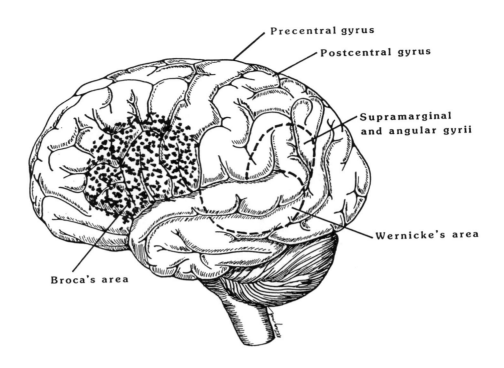

Precentral gyrus

Postcentral gyrus

Supramarginal
and angular gyrii

Wernicke's area

Broca's area

Impressions   Profound apraxia of speech/oral apraxia complex, associated with involvement of Areas 44 and 45, the motor strip and frontal eye field (Area 8) left cerebral hemisphere.

Discussion   Subsequent admitting CT scan proved negative, with MRI obtained approximately five days later showing a rather large left frontal lobe stroke. Given the findings of sinus tachycardia on EKG, it was believed that the patient's stroke was cardiogenic in origin. Because of concern for dysphagia, the patient underwent a videofluorographic study of swallow showing delayed oral preparation and transit, stasis of bolus material within the anterior oral cavity, delayed pharyngeal reflex, and premature swallow with approximately ten percent of the bolus material being aspirated. A reflexive cough was not elicited. Because of the concern for malnutrition as well as aspiration, a nasogastric feeding tube was placed subsequent to the swallowing study. Behavioral dysphagia therapy was implemented in conjunction with her speech therapy.

Because of the proximity of the lower motor (and sensory) strips to areas 44 and 45 (see illustration), it is not uncommon for patients with dyspraxia of speech to present with *central* facial and tongue weakness and limitation of movement. To what degree these neuromuscular signs adversely affect motor speech output, in the presence of overriding speech dyspraxia is difficult to determine. Treatment for this patient focused on the dyspraxic errors, along with facial and tongue exercises to improve strength and movement. Her motor speech remained essentially nonfunctional, although she could approximate "yes/no" and produce a number of isolated vowels or consonant-vowel combinations.

The patient's cardiac status remained stable during her stay on the Rehabilitation Unit. With time and therapy, she was able to take small amounts of thickened liquids and pureed solids, but remained on tube feedings for her primary source of nutrition. She continued to receive outpatient speech therapy and physical therapy for her right hemiparesis after discharge. Her left gaze preference eventually resolved.

10-Year-Old Female with Closed Head Injury and Language Disturbance

History   While riding home on her bicycle, this 10-year-old right-handed female was struck by an automobile. She was in a semicomatose state at the scene of the accident and was rushed to a trauma center.

Examination   On admission, her vital signs were normal, blood pressure was 130/70, pupils were equal, round, and reactive to light, and her neck was supple. Fractures of the wrist, ankle and eighth through twelfth thoracic ribs on the right side were detected. The right lower lung field had moderately reduced resonance to percussion, owing to puncture by one of the fractured ribs.

Multiple contusions were observed in areas of the head, face, chest, and limbs, most notably on the right side. Skull and cervical spine x-rays, however, revealed only those fractures described above. No sensory or motor deficiencies were detected in the limb or speech musculature. CT scan and EEG measurements were inconclusive. Her fractures and wounds were treated routinely, and she was admitted to hospital for further observation.

The patient was alert but periodically did not acknowledge her name. On occasion she could repeat two or three words in correct order. She variably recognized isolated letters but was unable to read or write to dictation. She could, however, copy various letters, words, and geometric shapes drawn by the examiner. She could not do simple mental calculations but accurately completed two paper-pencil computations.

When she spoke spontaneously, her speech was fluent, but plagued by disruptive jargon, neologistic distortion, and agrammatism. When asked to point to the ceiling, she said, "Sure! No! We're gonna mash it. One, two, three, I got it." She referred to her mother as her father and called a comb a brush. She periodically repeated portions of the alphabet and numbers 1 to 10 without provocation. Perseveration was evident on confrontation tasks.

Salient symptoms/signs	Test results	Impressions

This worksheet is to be used for recording relevant diagnostic observations. The blank illustration is to be used for identifying and sketching the suspected site of lesion(s). These steps should be completed prior to turning to the Impressions and illustrated site of lesion.

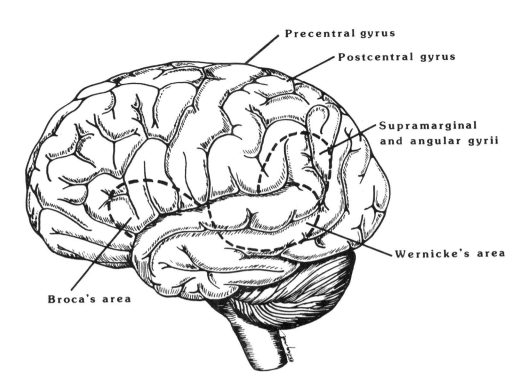

Precentral gyrus

Postcentral gyrus

Supramarginal
and angular gyrii

Wernicke's area

Broca's area

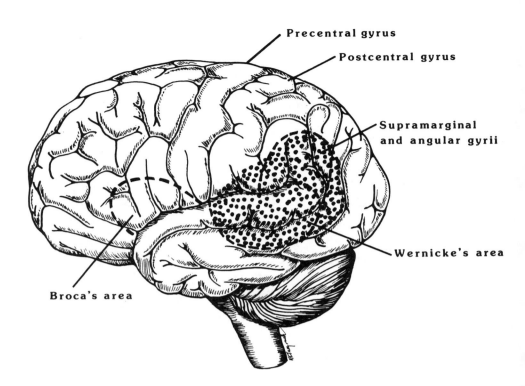

Precentral gyrus

Postcentral gyrus

Supramarginal
and angular gyrii

Wernicke's area

Broca's area

Impressions   Aphasia due to closed head injury.

Discussion   Nonpenetrating trauma to the skull is referred to as closed head injury. The symptoms caused by closed head trauma depend upon the regions of the brain damage and extent of injury. By inference, we felt that our patient sustained significant injury to the midtemporal-parietal and anterior occipital lobe area of the dominant hemisphere thus accounting for her language signs.

The term aphasia is frequently preceded by an adjective; that is, fluent, sensory, motor, and so forth. We prefer to use the term aphasia without a descriptor, in that on careful examination all the language modalities are involved to one degree or another. An adjective tells us little more than possibly the outstanding or principle presenting sign. The localizing value is debatable; the implications for treatment remain unclear.

Patients with aphasia have poor auditory-visual comprehension, although their expression may be articulate and fluent. The content may lack meaning resulting in empty speech, jargon, and neologisms.

The site of the lesion for aphasia is not neuroanatomically close to the origin and pathway of the pyramidal system; therefore, hemiplegia is not commonly associated with the disorder. Sensory signs may be recognized because of the proximity of the postcentral gyrus.

It is of interest to note that the patient's injuries were predominantly on the right side of her head and body, yet the speech-language signs were suggestive of a left hemisphere insult. This is presuming, of course, that she, like most people, is left-hemisphere-dominant for speech and language. Dominance should be established by age 10. A contrecoup injury can explain the signs: that is, the left side of the brain (opposite that which was struck) receives the brunt of the injury due to the brain's rebounding off the intracranial surface.

Patients who experience a single traumatic brain injury, who have no significant medical history, and who are young, seem to do well with therapy, and may experience full recovery.

59-Year-Old Female with History of Stroke Presents with Change in Speech

History   The patient is a 59-year-old female who was admitted to the emergency room following an acute onset of a change in speech on the evening prior to admission. There were no complaints of either weakness, numbness, clumsiness, visual changes, or difficulty swallowing. She did note, however, that she had some problem buttoning her blouse with her right hand.

Two years prior to admission, she had experienced a slight stroke that left her with mild residual right lower extremity weakness. She had a long history of hypertension, and was taking antihypertensive medications triamterene-hydrochlorothiazide (Dyazide) and metoprolol tartrate (Lopressor). She used tobacco and alcohol minimally. Her family history was negative for stroke, heart, or vascular disease.

Examination   The patient was cooperative and alert on examination. She was well oriented and in no apparent distress. Blood pressure was 142/78 and pulse was regular. Pupils were equal, round, and reactive to light. Visual fields were fully normal to confrontation. There was a question of mild flattening of the right nasolabial fold with preservation of the frontalis and orbital muscles on that side. Cranial nerves II through XII were intact bilaterally. With the exception of a question of mildly decreased sensation to pinprick in the right foot, and comparable right leg weakness, the remainder of the examination was normal. Cerebellar function was normal.

Once initiated, oral diadochokinetic rates were normal. Connected speech was marked by: (1) variable articulatory breakdown; (2) impaired intelligibility due to consonant and vowel addition, omission, substitution, and distortion; (3) repetition of sounds; and (4) articulatory groping. These error patterns worsened with increased speech length and complexity. Speaking rate was variably decreased in a manner that appeared to compensate for the articulatory imprecision.

Cough and hard glottal attack were sharp. Laryngeal function was within normal limits; there were no resonatory or respiratory findings. Assessment of language function revealed all auditory, visual, naming, and calculation tasks to be within normal limits. During writing tasks occasionally a word was misspelled or a letter transposed; these errors were frequently self-corrected. Although she was rather anxious during the examination, both the patient and her spouse indicated that this was her usual state.

Salient symptoms/signs	Test results	Impressions

This worksheet is to be used for recording relevant diagnostic observations. The blank illustration is to be used for identifying and sketching the suspected site of lesion(s). These steps should be completed prior to turning to the Impressions and illustrated site of lesion.

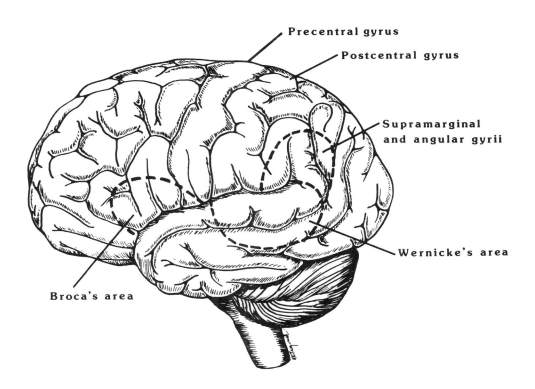

Precentral gyrus

Postcentral gyrus

Supramarginal
and angular gyrii

Wernicke's area

Broca's area

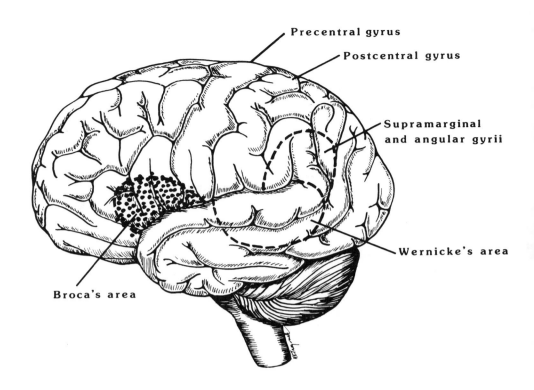

Precentral gyrus

Postcentral gyrus

Supramarginal
and angular gyrii

Wernicke's area

Broca's area

Impressions   Apraxia of speech, secondary to left cerebral hemisphere stroke.

Discussion   Both EEG and CT scan were normal. Angiography revealed bilateral internal carotid artery ulcerations and plaques, greater on the left than on the right. She underwent a left carotid endarterectomy for correction of the stenosis one week following initial admission.

The nature of apraxia of speech is an ongoing controversy. It is viewed by many as a motor speech planning disorder, which frequently co-occurs with oral apraxia, characterized by difficulty planning non-speech acts, such as lip pursing, wiggling of the tongue, and so on. Interestingly, this was not observed in our patient.

Speech apraxia is characterized by many of the signs demonstrated by our patient, including sound omissions, transpositions and additions, and articulatory groping. The rate, or prosodic modification, is thought to be either a compensatory part of the disorder as the patient attempts to modify the articulatory imprecision, or an inherent part of the disorder itself. Many believe that the signs are consistent with what has been called expressive, Broca's, or nonfluent aphasia, and, historically, cortical dysarthria. The former terms, however, imply that the disorder may be language- rather than speech-based, thereby propagating the disagreement.

The occurrence of apraxia of speech in isolation is not common; it typically cooccurs with (1) contralateral corticobulbar and corticospinal tract (upper motor neuron) signs, and (2) aphasia. With the exception of a question of a mild right central facial paresis and right extremity weakness (which may have been residuals of an earlier stroke) there were no indications of upper motor neuron involvement in this presentation. Differential diagnosis was further confounded by normal EEG and CT scan. In the latter measurement, however, a recent stroke may not be detected until approximately three to five days after the event; and if small enough, possibly never.

Co-occurring dressing apraxia is frequently seen in frontal lobe involvement. Dysgraphia does occur with dyspraxia of speech and frequently mirrors the articulation and prosodic deficits. This was true for our patient.

The patient was seen for speech therapy following endarterectomy and regained many of her premorbid speaking skills. She was placed on dipyridamole (Persantine) and received outpatient speech therapy. One-year follow-up examination, including carotid ultrasound, revealed minor calcium plaques in both common carotid arteries without obstructed flow. CT scan remained normal. However, it was the clinical consensus that the site of lesion responsible for the speech and motor signs was in Broca's region (Brodmann's area 44) of the left cerebral hemisphere.

case 64

9-Year-Old Male with History of Fever and Delirium Has Inattentiveness, Poor Grades, Drowsiness, and Speech Disturbance

History A 9-year-old male had been hospitalized for a fever in excess of 100 degrees and delirium, which had persisted for 17 hours. During the next week, he experienced an increased pulse rate, joint pain, chills, and continued fever, restlessness and occasional and mild auditory and visual hallucinations. He was treated symptomatically with alcohol and warm sponge baths to reduce the temperature. Toward the end of the week, the temperature dropped rapidly to within normal limits, leaving him somnolent and mildly confused.

Following discharge from the hospital, the patient continued to complain of fatigue, and his parents felt he was somewhat irritable and restless. His grades in school dropped and his teachers noted inattentiveness, poor behavior, and clumsiness particularly of the upper limbs. His speech seemed slurred and imprecise.

Examination Clinical examination was remarkable for quick, irregular, jerky movements of the upper extremities, head, and facies that were present at rest and exacerbated during movement. Rapid alternating hand movements rendered similar results with occasional overflow (abnormal movements in another part of the body) to the face. Overflow was also apparent when the patient was asked to grab the examiner's hand. Muscles were moderately weak without atrophy or tenderness, and reflexes brisk. Attempts to elicit a reflex frequently resulted in overflow.

The tongue would not remain at midline on protrusion; quick asynchronous movements of the soft palate and posterior pharyngeal wall were noted on depression of the mandible. The lips could not be maintained in a pursed posture without similar interruptive and uncontrollable movements.

Articulation was characterized by moderately irregular breakdown of articulatory precision in connected speech. Oral alternate and sequential motion rates were moderately irregular. Vocal quality was mildly harsh with occasional voice arrests on vowel prolongation. Speaking rate was variably fast-slow with occasional inappropriate silences within sentences.

Salient symptoms/signs	Test results	Impressions

This worksheet is to be used for recording relevant diagnostic observations. The blank illustration is to be used for identifying and sketching the suspected site of lesion(s). These steps should be completed prior to turning to the Impressions and illustrated site of lesion.

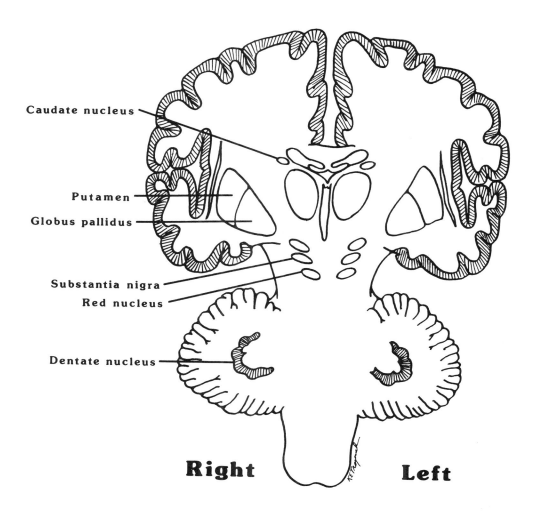

Caudate nucleus

Putamen

Globus pallidus

Substantia nigra

Red nucleus

Dentate nucleus

Right　　　**Left**

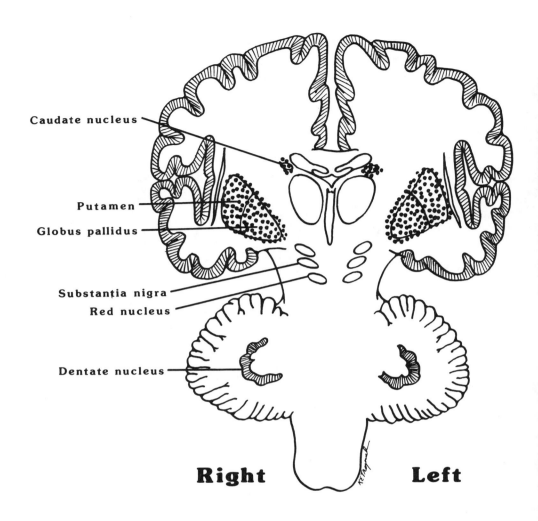

Caudate nucleus

Putamen

Globus pallidus

Substanția nigra

Red nucleus

Dentate nucleus

Right

Left

Impressions Hyperkinetic (quick) dysarthria of Sydenham's chorea.

Discussion The patient's clinical history suggests that his movement disorder was precipitated by rheumatic fever. One sequela to this condition is *Sydenham's chorea,* which is characterized by very quick, jerky, involuntary, and irregular movements of the limbs and orofacial musculature. Occurring in youngsters, this condition implicates disturbances in basal ganglia functioning, not unlike the pathophysiology of Huntington's disease. Whereas the latter condition is familial, occurs between the third and fifth decade, and is ultimately fatal, the symptoms and signs of Sydenham's chorea usually subside within two to three months.

When speech musculature are involved, a quick form of hyperkinetic dysarthria results. The articulation, phonation, and prosodic disturbances exhibited by our patient are typical features.

Treatment of Sydenham's chorea may consist of bed rest and mild doses of sedatives such as phenobarbitol or tranquilizers such as phenothiazines or haloperidol (Haldol). Corticosteroids may further help reduce the effects and recurrence of rheumatic fever. At the time of this report, four months postonset, the patient was doing well and his speech had improved significantly.

51-Year-Old Female with Abnormal Voice

History The patient is a 51-year-old, left-handed Laotian female with no formal education. She came to the United States fifteen years ago and was originally seen by an internist for evaluation of atypical chest pain. Subsequent evaluations including echocardiography, blood gas, pulmonary, and thyroid function studies proved normal. She had a depressed affect and was hoarse. The patient did not speak English; therefore, the examination was undertaken through an interpreter. The patient readily admitted to being depressed for a number of years in that she felt she did not have enough children (she was the mother of four) and that her oldest son had been with a gang and in trouble with the law. She associated the onset of her hoarseness with the discovery of her son's gang activities approximately five years before being seen. She was referred to psychiatry, where she was started on antidepressant medication that proved to have little effect on her depression and no influence on her voice.

Her voice symptoms had not progressed, although they worsened when she was depressed or anxious. She had never experienced total voice loss or difficulty swallowing or breathing or instances of nasal reflux. She felt that there was a "gap" in her voice. She had no other concerns about her speech, language, or cognition. Since onset, her voice had never returned to normal.

There were no complaints for vision or gait. She had noted some shakiness of the right upper extremity during manual activities. There were no changes in muscle bulk or strength and no cramping. The family history was negative for a communicative, cognitive, or movement disorder. She was not taking prescribed medication at the time of examination. She did not use ethanol or tobacco.

Examination Examination revealed an affectively depressed patient who was periodically tearful and had only fleeting eye contact with the examiner. The structural integrity of the speech mechanism was sound for speech production, while cranial nerves V (motor and sensory), VII, and IX through XII were clinically functioning within normal limits. There were no pathologic reflexes. With the exception of the phonatory/laryngeal signs, the remainder of the motor speech examination was within normal limits.

Conversational speech and vowel prolongation were characterized by mild/moderate hoarse-breathy dysphonia on a standard rating scale. She would not perform during maximum phonation testing, indicating that she felt embarrassed because of her voice. However, on brief vowel prolongation, there were instances of regular changes in volume at modal and high modal registers, estimated to be between 4 and 6 Hz, with occasional superimposed adductor voice arrest (laryngeal spasm). Rigid laryngeal endoscopy confirmed regular and rhythmic movements of the true and false vocal folds, with cessation of phonation when the folds were in the adducted position. The signs were further delineated by laryngeal stroboscopy.

Through an interpreter, there were no gross signs of language or cognitive involvement.

Salient symptoms/signs	Test results	Impressions

This worksheet is to be used for recording relevant diagnostic observations. The blank illustration is to be used for identifying and sketching the suspected site of lesion(s). These steps should be completed prior to turning to the Impressions and illustrated site of lesion.

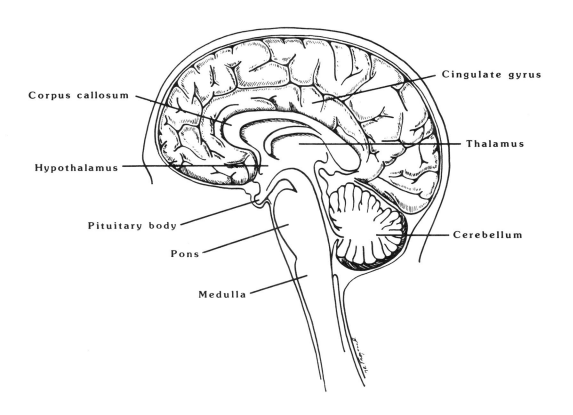

Corpus callosum

Cingulate gyrus

Hypothalamus

Thalamus

Pituitary body

Pons

Cerebellum

Medulla

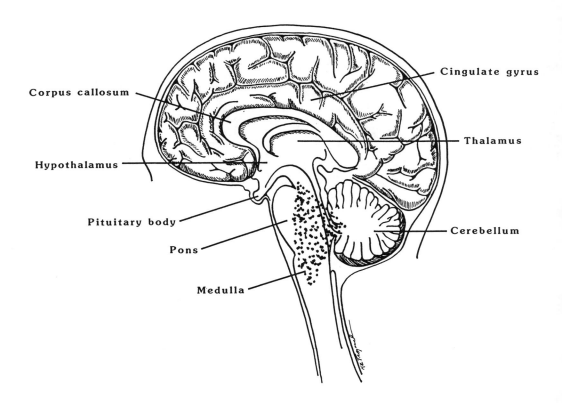

Impressions   Mild essential (voice) tremor as a component of essential tremor syndrome or early adductor spastic (spasmodic) dysphonia of essential tremor.

Discussion   After further discussion and investigation into the patient's history, it became apparent that, indeed, her voice change coincided roughly with the time her eldest son became involved in gang activities, which had placed significant stress on the family, in general, and the patient, specifically. The situation was exacerbated by the pressure and negativism that the Hmong community placed on her because of her son's antisocial activities.

The patient was referred to a neurologist, who identified a postural tremor of the right upper extremity. At the time of this report, a pharmacologic regimen had been outlined that would include a trial of propranolol (Inderal), primidone (Mysoline), or methazolamide (Neptazane). She was not felt to be a candidate for botulinum toxin injection therapy at that time. Moreover, based on the standards of her culture, the patient was obligated to consult with the community shaman before undergoing any medical therapy.

This patient demonstrated psychopathologic illness in conjunction with a neurogenic voice disorder, the former most likely precipitating the latter—a finding that is not uncommon in neurology, particularly as it relates to the onset of certain movement disorders. In most instances of the type of voice tremor described here, the neuroanatomic site of lesion is not evident with imaging studies, although the brainstem pathways outlined in the figure are often implicated.

75-Year-Old Male with Progressive Symptoms, Including Deterioration in Strength, Swallowing, and Speech

History The patient is a 75-year-old right-handed male referred for evaluation of progressive weakness for approximately six months, weight loss of 50 pounds, and constipation. He also reported increased fatigability and periodic difficulty swallowing. These symptoms were preceded by progressive deterioration in speech and gait for approximately two years. Interestingly, his father, older brothers, and two sisters had similar symptoms. He denied changes in language function, exposure to toxins, illness, infections; nor had he experienced traumatic injury. During the present hospitalization he was found to have anemia and pleural effusion.

Examination On examination, the patient was awake, alert, and well oriented. Pupils were reactive; some right gaze nystagmus was noted; hearing was judged normal, as were all cranial nerves. The gag reflex was considered brisk. A course tremor, greater on the left than on the right, was noted on finger-to-nose testing. Deep tendon reflexes were brisk, but symmetrical. Gait was unsteady. CT scan suggested cerebellar degeneration, with normal cerebral hemispheres.

The facial musculature appeared hypotonic. Palmomental, sucking, and jaw-jerk reflexes were elicited. Articulation in connected speech was marked by variable articulatory breakdown, which moderately impaired intelligibility. Oral diadochokinetic and sequential motion rates were slow and imprecise. Phonation was marked by continued breathiness, with intermittent and variable harsh to strained-strangled quality. These signs were most evident during contextual speech and vowel prolongation. Periodically, the patient's voice lapsed into a "wail."

Cough and hard glottal attack were considered mildly reduced. Indirect rigid laryngoscopic examination revealed mild, incomplete, but symmetrical vocal fold adduction and abduction. Intermittent hypernasality and nasal emission, along with decreased speaking rate and prolonged intervals between utterances, were evident. Respiratory support for speech was forced and somewhat effortful.

Salient symptoms/signs	Test results	Impressions

This worksheet is to be used for recording relevant diagnostic observations. The blank illustration is to be used for identifying and sketching the suspected site of lesion(s). These steps should be completed prior to turning to the Impressions and illustrated site of lesion.

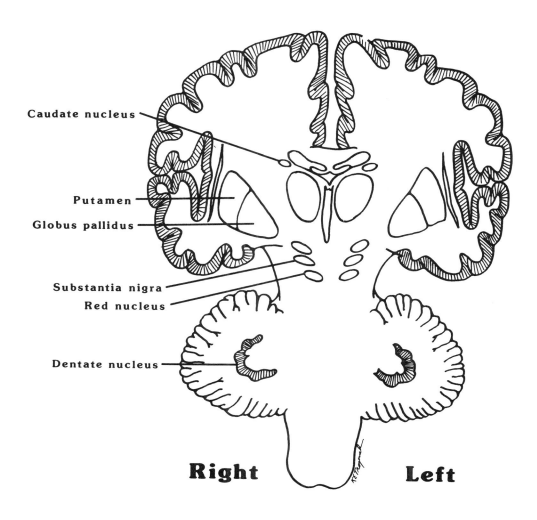

Caudate nucleus

Putamen

Globus pallidus

Substantia nigra

Red nucleus

Dentate nucleus

Right　　　　**Left**

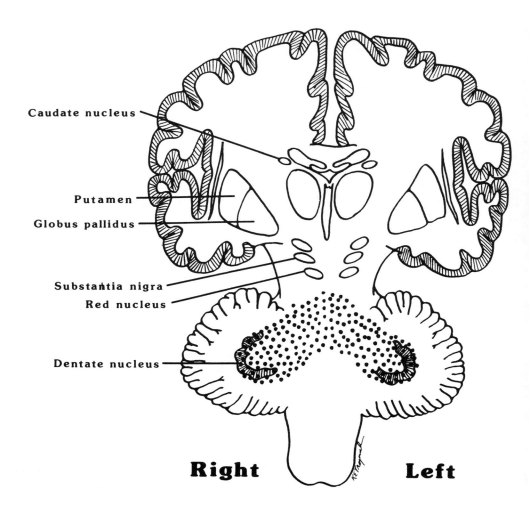

Caudate nucleus

Putamen

Globus pallidus

Substantia nigra

Red nucleus

Dentate nucleus

Right

Left

75-Year-Old Male with Progressive Symptoms, Including Deterioration in Strength, Swallowing, and Speech

Impressions   Mixed spastic-ataxic dysarthria owing to idiopathic familial cerebellar (olivoponto-cerebellar) degeneration.

Discussion   This patient presented a rather interesting clinical picture. The majority of his limb and truncal signs, including the course bilateral upper extremity tremor and gait difficulties, were consistent with cerebellar disease. The preponderance of motor speech findings, however, were consistent with bilateral corticobulbar tract damage and resultant spastic dysarthria. The grossly imprecise oral alternate motion rates and possibly vocal harshness suggested cerebellar involvement and ataxic dysarthria.

The genesis of this patient's swallowing difficulty is rather interesting diagnostically. As he ate both liquids and solids, neuromotor discoordination resulted in rather awkward posterior movement of the bolus. The beginning of the reflexive phase of swallowing was then marked by discoordinated oropharyngeal movements that caused pooling around and leakage through the laryngeal vestibule. The aspiration (albeit minimal) that occurred was likely due to laryngeal hypotonia.

Fortunately for this patient, the progression of neurologic symptoms and signs has been rather insidious. It is conceivable, however, that at some time he may need a tracheostomy and possibly an alternate means of feeding as the signs progress. He is currently able to express himself verbally, albeit with some difficulty and impaired intelligibility. He is being considered for an augmentative (nonverbal) communication system.

Like many of the cerebellar and spinocerebellar degeneration syndromes, the cause of this particular familial disorder has not been determined. It is, however, thought to be autosomal dominant in nature.

15-Year-Old Male with Progressive Incoordination, Tremor, and Speech Disturbance

History A previously healthy 15-year-old male began experiencing weakness, tremor, and incoordination of the head and limbs during various activities. Since his prior medical history was unremarkable and he had been under considerable academic and familial stress, his symptoms were judged to be psychogenic phenomena and counseling was recommended. However, the difficulties slowly progressed over the next year, necessitating referral by the family physician to a neurologist.

Neurological examination revealed incoordination of gait, slow and irregular alternate motion rates of the limbs, and slight intention tremor of the head and arms. The signs suggested the possibility of cerebellar dysfunction, but a definitive diagnosis could not be made. There was no familial history of a similar movement disorder. All laboratory studies including CT scan were normal. The patient was scheduled to return for a reevaluation in six months. Three months later, however, he began experiencing episodes of nausea, vomiting, and slurring of speech; and his arms and legs felt weaker.

Examination All limbs were hypotonic with muscle strength slightly reduced. Gait was jerky, unsteady, and wide-based; alternate motion rates of the upper limbs were slow and irregular. Mild intention tremor of the head and arms was also evident. CT scan now showed degenerative cerebellar changes.

The facies appeared normal. Isolated pursing, puckering, and smiling movements of the lips were performed without difficulty. Alternate and sequential movements of the lips, however, were imprecise, slower than normal, and irregular in timing. The tongue had a hypotonic appearance at rest, but there were no signs of atrophy or fasciculations; decreased resistance to passive movement was also noted. Isolated movements in all directions were within normal limits, although alternate and sequential movements were slow, imprecise, and irregular.

Articulation was variably slow, scanning, and imprecise; it sounded as if the patient was intoxicated. Intervals between words were occasionally prolonged, as were sounds within words. Vowel prolongation was slightly tremulous, while contextual speech was marked by harsh quality with an overlay of monoloud and monopitch characteristics. Resonance and respiratory support for speech were felt to be normal and adequate.

Salient symptoms/signs	Test results	Impressions

This worksheet is to be used for recording relevant diagnostic observations. The blank illustration is to be used for identifying and sketching the suspected site of lesion(s). These steps should be completed prior to turning to the Impressions and illustrated site of lesion.

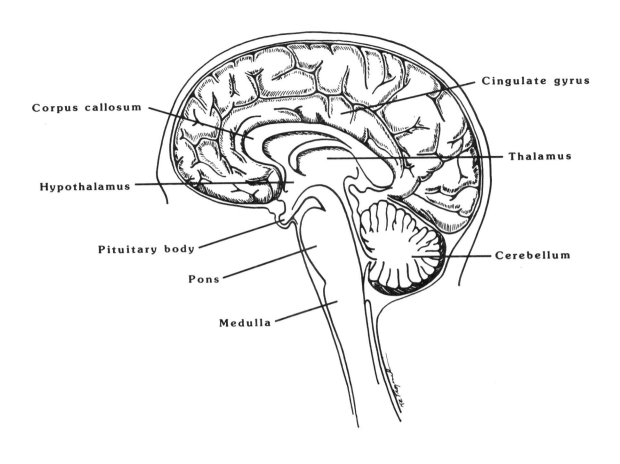

Corpus callosum

Cingulate gyrus

Hypothalamus

Thalamus

Pituitary body

Cerebellum

Pons

Medulla

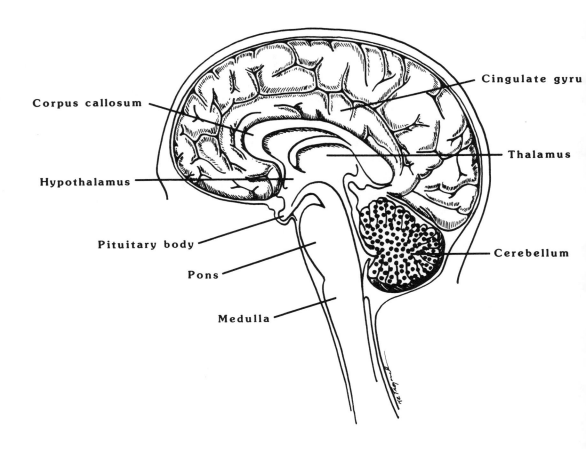

Corpus callosum

Cingulate gyru

Thalamus

Hypothalamus

Pituitary body

Pons

Cerebellum

Medulla

Impressions   Ataxic dysarthria and generalized dyssynergia.

Discussion   The signs and symptoms of this case were manifestations of idiopathic, progressive, and degenerative cerebellar disease. Normally, the cerebellum aids in the balance, coordination, integration, rhythm, timing, speed, and force of all muscular contractions. Diffuse or multifocal cerebellar lesions or involvement of cerebellar pathways usually result in failure of one or more of these functions. The terms *dyssynergia* or *dysmetria* are used, in a generic sense, to refer to such failures.

Unilateral cerebellar hemisphere damage produces ipsilateral skeletal signs. Left cerebellar hemisphere involvement may produce a dysarthria because of crossed supratentorial tracts and the prosodic control features of the right cerebral hemisphere. Right cerebellar damage may spare speech. Bilateral or midline involvement adversely affects the head, neck, and truncal musculature, as well as producing a dysarthria, as observed in this case.

Head movements and posturing are incoordinated, and walking is characterized by an unsteady, reeling, and wide-based posture, commonly referred to as cerebellar gait or ataxia. Vertigo and nausea are secondary conditions that typically accompany the ataxia. Because of the proximity to and complex relationship with the pyramidal tract, corticospinal and corticobulbar signs may be identified in cerebellar diseases. Ataxic dysarthria is rather distinct perceptually. Patients sound inebriated, primarily because of prolongation of words and intervals between words; excess stress on normally unstressed words; and slow, imprecise, and irregularly timed articulation.

20-Year-Old Male with Head Injury and Language Disturbance

History   The patient is a 20-year-old male who was involved in a motor vehicle accident on the day of admission. He was semiconscious at the scene of the accident. On admission to the emergency room, his responses to verbal commands were inappropriate and accompanied by grunting and groaning. Strength was decreased bilaterally, more so on the right. He was hyperreflexive bilaterally and had numerous contusions and lacerations. Admitting CT scan revealed a large intratemporal hematoma in the left cerebral hemisphere. The patient was taken immediately to surgery for evacuation of the lesion. Following surgery and a period of convalescence, he was admitted to the rehabilitation service for comprehensive evaluation and treatment.

Examination   On examination the patient was alert, although somewhat restless. There was moderate weakness in the upper and lower extremities bilaterally, but greater on the right side; a Babinski response was elicited on that side. The deep tendon reflexes were brisk bilaterally but greater on the right. He neglected the right visual field. There were no other sensory findings. Neuromuscular speech functioning was normal.

The patient exhibited marked auditory and visual comprehension deficits, as well as short-term memory difficulties on simple and complex tasks. Visual stimuli had to be presented in the left visual field to be seen and comprehended. He frequently misnamed common objects and pictures, although when he verbally rehearsed before responding, his answers were considerably more accurate.

He was frequently perseverative and occasionally neologistic. He variably recognized these errors. The majority of items requiring mental and paper-pencil calculations were missed. Written response to dictation was poor orthographically because of the weak preferred upper extremity. He was able to copy shapes and letters accurately, however. The patient was oriented to time, place, and person, although his responses were abbreviated.

Salient symptoms/signs	Test results	Impressions

This worksheet is to be used for recording relevant diagnostic observations. The blank illustration is to be used for identifying and sketching the suspected site of lesion(s). These steps should be completed prior to turning to the Impressions and illustrated site of lesion.

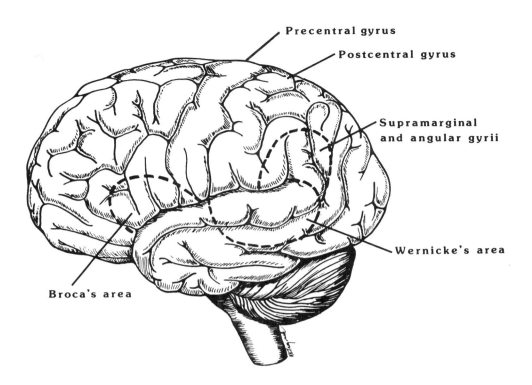

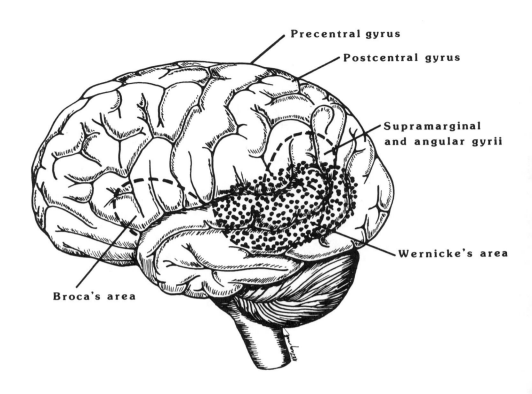

Impressions   Aphasia due to traumatic head injury and intracerebral hematoma.

Discussion   A typical sequela to head injury is diffuse or multifocal brain pathology. This results in a matrix of behavioral and cognitive signs that have been described as confusion or confused language. Along with the trauma itself, the cause of confused language is considered to include contrecoup injury, whereby a blow to the head causes the brain to rebound off the opposite inner wall of the skull. It is somewhat unusual to see a relatively focal communicative deficit (that is, aphasia) following closed head trauma. It is conceivable that our patient's aphasia evolved from more widespread cognitive deficits.

The bilateral weakness, greater on the right, suggests bilateral corticospinal tract damage, possibly greater on the left. This was further substantiated by the Babinski sign and brisk reflexes on the right. Right side neglect, which frequently includes homonymous hemianopsia, suggests involvement beyond the optic chiasm, particularly the left parietal-occipital zone and associated optic radiations. These cortical and subcortical areas are chief components of the visual pathways from the left temporal and right nasal retina. It could be argued that both the motor and visual signs were secondary to the generalized brain injury and the edema surrounding the hematoma.

The patient received concentrated speech therapy and recovered a majority of his premorbid communicative skills. In general, patients with traumatically induced aphasia experience greater recovery of language skills than do those whose disorder is secondary to infarction or neoplasm.

60-Year-Old Female with Progressive Deterioration of Speech and Swallowing

History A 60-year-old female with a long history of hypertension began experiencing progressive deterioration of speech and swallowing over several months. She had difficulty eating both liquid and solid foods because of episodic choking. She was periodically embarrassed by drooling while eating, speaking, and while at rest. Although she was ambulatory, she remarked that her legs felt weak and heavy.

Examination On clinical neurologic testing deep tendon reflexes in the lower limbs were brisk and muscle strength was mildly reduced; upper limb reflexes were mildly brisk while strength seemed unimpaired. The face looked weak in repose; sucking, jaw-jerk, and palmomental reflex were elicited. Movements of the lips during puckering, smiling, and diadochokinetic tasks were reduced in range, slow-labored, and a moderate degree of weakness of the lips was evident.

The tongue was anatomically intact; however, protrusion, depression, elevation, and lateralization were limited in range. Anterior and lateral tongue strength were moderately reduced. Movements during lingual diadochokinetic tasks were slow-labored and imprecise. The velum was symmetrical at rest and during production of a neutral vowel; however, posterior superior movement was slow. The gag reflex was brisk.

Language skills were normal. Articulation was mildly slow-labored, and imprecise. Errors primarily consisted of distortions of consonants. Voice was mildly strained-strangled and monopitched with intermittent phonatory arrests. Periodic hypernasal resonance and snorting were also noted, which added to the speech deficit. Videofluorographic study of the swallow revealed increased time from the oral through the pharyngeal stages and pooling at the level of the valecula with resultant aspiration.

CT scan suggested at least two hypodense lesions involving the internal capsule. Cerebral angiography revealed atherosclerotic changes in both the internal carotid arteries, particularly at the bifurcations.

Salient symptoms/signs	Test results	Impressions

This worksheet is to be used for recording relevant diagnostic observations. The blank illustration is to be used for identifying and sketching the suspected site of lesion(s). These steps should be completed prior to turning to the Impressions and illustrated site of lesion.

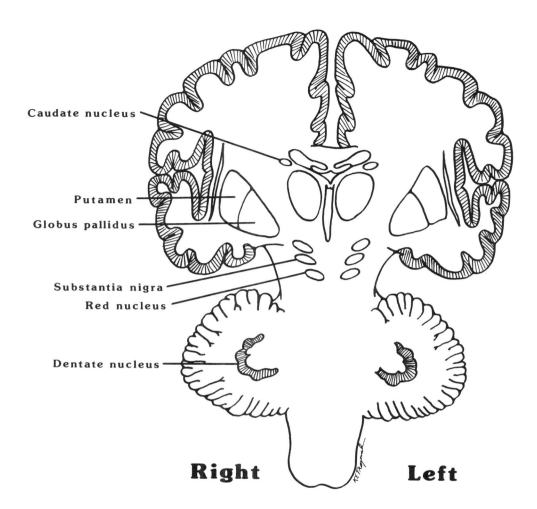

Caudate nucleus

Putamen

Globus pallidus

Substantia nigra

Red nucleus

Dentate nucleus

Right   **Left**

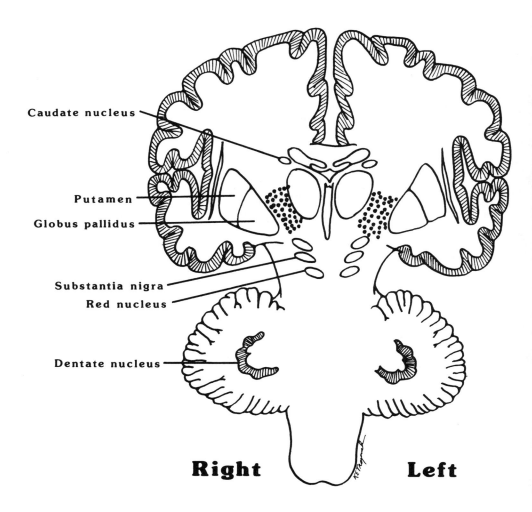

Caudate nucleus

Putamen

Globus pallidus

Substantia nigra

Red nucleus

Dentate nucleus

Right

Left

Impressions   Spastic dysarthria.

Discussion   The signs and symptoms of this case support the diagnosis of spastic (bilateral upper motor neuron) dysarthria most likely secondary to infarcts involving the corticobulbar and corticospinal tracts at the level of the internal capsules. The dysphagia and drooling were felt to be manifestations of impaired movement and weakness of the speech and swallowing musculature.

The CT scan and angiography provided a rather straightforward diagnosis in this case. Clinically, hypertensive patients are at high risk for small vessel disease. Our patient's findings were consistent with distal middle cerebral artery involvement. The lenticular striate perforating branches of this artery supply a good portion of the internal capsule. Strokes in this area are sometimes referred to as capsular or lacunar infarcts, with the resultant signs being primarily motor than sensory.

History   A 41-year-old college instructor, with a history of periodic headache and blurred vision, was referred for a neurologic evaluation by an ophthalmologist who noted papilledema on examination for eyeglasses. For the past year she had been experiencing eye strain when reading at night. With the exception of the eye findings, the clinical neurologic examination was well within normal limits.

A CT scan of the head revealed an enhancing mass in the right frontal region with considerable edema of the right frontal lobe suggestive of an olfactory groove lesion, possibly meningioma. The patient was admitted to the hospital for further evaluation.

Following angiography, the patient suffered dense right hemiplegia, right homonymous hemianopsia, and mutism. Within three days of angiography she showed improved neurologic function on the right side and clearing of the right visual field defect. A significant communication disorder remained, however. Serial CT scans showed little reduction in the edema involving the right frontal lobe, despite 10 days of corticosteroid treatment.

The lesion, which proved to be a meningioma, was excised and gross total removal was accomplished. The postoperative course was uncomplicated, and the patient was discharged eight days following the procedure. Follow-up consultation was sought in neurology and speech pathology.

Examination   With the exception of the mild residual right hemiparesis, with the arm involved more than the leg, and comparable right central facial paresis marked by flattening of the nasolabial fold, the neurologic examination was not impressive. Visual fields were now well within normal limits.

Examination of motor speech function revealed mild imprecision of bilabial consonants (/**p**/ and /**b**/) secondary to the facial weakness on the right. Phonation was mildly breathy with decreased volume and a somewhat hoarse quality. The patient indicated, however, that this was "normal for me." Oral diadochokinetic and sequential motion rates were mildly slow and comparably irregular.

Nonspeech oral volitional movements were marked by 41 percent error, while production of multisyllabic words and complex sentences was characterized by articulatory groping, sound and syllable transposition, and difficulty with sound initiation. These difficulties adversely affected prosody (speaking rhythm): the patient either tried to compensate for or anticipate these errors. Both resonation and respiration were considered adequate for speech.

Although the patient adequately followed simple conversation, 30 percent of the items requiring knowledge of right-left orientation, 10 percent of the items requiring comprehension of one-step commands, and 60 percent of the items requiring comprehension of two-step complex commands were missed. She also missed 30 percent of the items requiring knowledge of prepositions and spatial relationships; that is, on, under, away from, and the like.

Auditory retention was considered somewhat reduced; she retained 4 digits forward and 11 syllables and 9 words. It is conceivable that her speech deficit interfered with performance on this task. Of the items used to assess visual comprehension, 30 percent were missed. Of items to be named, 13 percent were missed. She was frequently perseverative on this task. Ninety percent of the items requiring mental calculation following a verbal stimulus, and 40 percent of the items requiring paper-pencil computation were missed. Using the preferred right upper extremity, she was able to copy orthographic symbols accurately, but missed 50 percent of the items requiring a written response to dictation.

Worksheet

Salient symptoms/signs	Test results	Impressions

This worksheet is to be used for recording relevant diagnostic observations. The blank illustration is to be used for identifying and sketching the suspected site of lesion(s). These steps should be completed prior to turning to the Impressions and illustrated site of lesion.

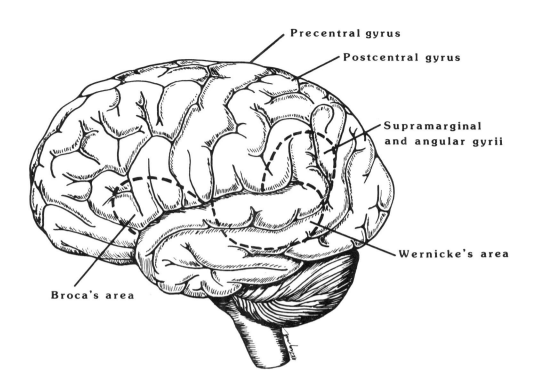

Precentral gyrus

Postcentral gyrus

Supramarginal
and angular gyrii

Wernicke's area

Broca's area

423   *41-Year-Old Female with History of Headache and Blurred Vision Has Language and Speech Disturbances Following Angiography*

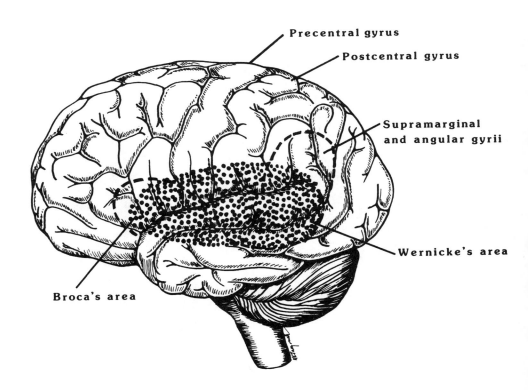

Precentral gyrus

Postcentral gyrus

Supramarginal
and angular gyrii

Wernicke's area

Broca's area

41-Year-Old Female with History of Headache and Blurred Vision Has Language and Speech Disturbances Following Angiography

Impressions   Moderate speech/oral apraxia with comparable aphasia, consistent with involvement of the left cerebral hemisphere.

Discussion   This patient's history highlights the potential hazards associated with certain diagnostic procedures—in her case, angiography. Such complications fortunately are rather rare in comparison to the number of procedures done. Further benefits of such diagnostic procedures usually outweigh the possible liabilities.

It is evident from the history that our patient experienced a rather significant ictus (sudden event) following angiography. A follow-up CT scan three weeks after discharge revealed: (1) almost complete resolution of the edema of the right hemisphere following removal of the meningioma; and (2) a zone of diminished density in the left frontal-temporal region, consistent with infarction, which was considered iatrogenic (induced by treatment) in origin secondary to angiography.

The patient's right hemiplegia and central facial paresis suggest involvement of the left corticospinal and corticobulbar tracts, respectively. Her apraxic and aphasic signs were consistent with the involvement of the left frontal-temporal zones identified on the CT scans.

The patient received concentrated outpatient speech therapy for approximately two months and regained skills in both speech and language that allowed her to return to her vocation as a college instructor. Her standards for communicative effectiveness and the requirements of the teaching profession no doubt were important motivational stimuli in the recovery process.

56-Year-Old Male with Progressive Weakness, Cramping of the Limbs, and Deterioration of Speech and Swallowing

History   A 56-year-old truck driver was forced to retire early because of progressive weakening and cramping of his arms, hands, and legs over the course of two years. According to his spouse, shortly after his retirement, he began to regurgitate liquids through his nose, choke on foods, demonstrate slurred speech, and was forced to use a cane because of his leg weakness.

Examination   Throughout testing, he was alert and cooperative although periodically emotionally labile. His use of language was judged to be age-appropriate. Significant test findings included the following: (1) bilateral exaggerated deep tendon reflexes of the upper and lower limbs; (2) atrophy and fasciculations of the intrinsic muscles of the hands; (3) moderate to severe weakness of the upper and lower limbs, with associated bilateral Babinski signs; (4) atrophy and weakness of the left half of the tongue and face; (5) during vowel prolongation, symmetrical but reduced velopharyngeal function without evidence of atrophy; (6) a hyperactive gag reflex; (7) mild to moderate articulatory imprecision; (8) severe variable hypernasal resonance and nasal emission; (9) strained-strangled phonation with intermittent periods of wet-gurgly hoarseness; (10) decreased volitional cough and weak vocal cord approximation on direct laryngoscopy; and (11) moderately reduced lingual and labial alternate motion rates.

EMG showed diffuse degeneration of motor units of the upper and lower limbs. CT scans, myelograms, and brainstem auditory-evoked responses proved normal.

Salient symptoms/signs	Test results	Impressions

This worksheet is to be used for recording relevant diagnostic observations. The blank illustration is to be used for identifying and sketching the suspected site of lesion(s). These steps should be completed prior to turning to the Impressions and illustrated site of lesion.

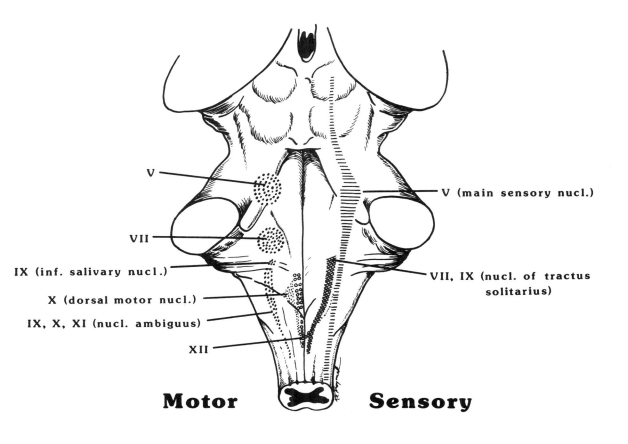

V

VII

IX (inf. salivary nucl.)

X (dorsal motor nucl.)

IX, X, XI (nucl. ambiguus)

XII

V (main sensory nucl.)

VII, IX (nucl. of tractus solitarius)

Motor   **Sensory**

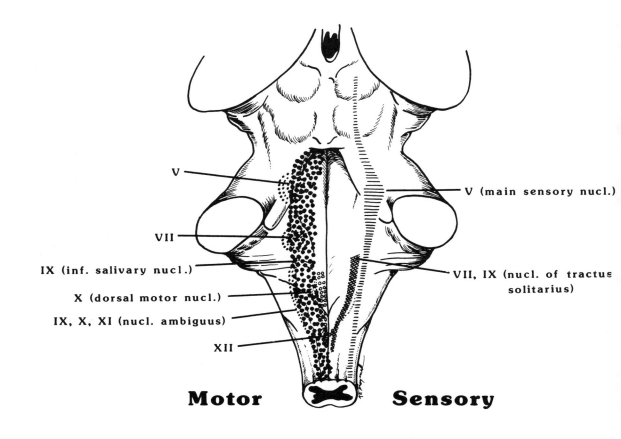

V

V (main sensory nucl.)

VII

IX (inf. salivary nucl.)

X (dorsal motor nucl.)

IX, X, XI (nucl. ambiguus)

XII

VII, IX (nucl. of tractus
solitarius)

Motor   **Sensory**

Impressions   Mixed flaccid-spastic dysarthria, caused by a slowly progressive course of amyotrophic lateral sclerosis (ALS).

Discussion   ALS is one of many progressive and fatal neurologic diseases involving both upper and lower motor neurons. The etiology of this disease remains unclear. Although the average course of the illness is approximately three years, some individuals with a slowly progressive form may live as long as 10 or more years. When bulbar signs are presenting features, the longevity is shortened, the patient frequently succumbing to aspiration pneumonia.

The dysarthria of ALS is typically characterized by imprecise articulation, hypernasality, variable wet-hoarse and strained-strangled phonation, and reduced control of pitch and loudness variations. Speech and swallowing disturbances are caused by widespread weakness, paralysis, incoordination, and altered tone of the muscles of the face, tongue, velopharynx, and larynx.

The dysphagia in our patient suggests problems with oral transit as well as pharyngeal-laryngeal control, which are most likely secondary to upper and lower motor neuron involvement. Likewise, speech signs implicate select cranial nerves and the corticobulbar tracts.

The hyperreflexive deep tendon responses and bilateral Babinski signs implicate the corticospinal tracts. The atrophy and fasciculations of the hands suggest anterior horn cell (cervical spinal nerve, LMN) involvement, and the associated weakness may be secondary to both UMN and LMN degeneration. In suspected cases of motor neuron disease EMG is tantamount to accurate diagnosis.

Treatment of patients with ALS is palliative and may involve: (1) tracheostomy; (2) altered feeding, such as gastrostomy; and (3) augmentative (nonverbal) communication as the disease progresses.

47-Year-Old Male with Closed Head Injury

History   The patient is a 47-year-old male who was in good health until attacked by two men with baseball bats. He was found in a semiconscious state and taken to a hospital by ambulance. In the ER, the patient was unable to answer specific questions about the events leading to the injury, but did recall being attacked by two men. Skull films and MRI of the head revealed crushing skull base and suture line fractures of the left temporal and occipital bones, with mild inflammatory changes involving the left middle and superior temporal lobe gyri, associated with regional subdural edema, respectively. The patient was admitted for observation and evaluation.

Examination   On examination, the patient was somewhat lethargic but alert and well-oriented to general events and surroundings. There were no focal language or neurocognitive signs. Assessment of speech revealed moderate degrees of (1) hypernasal resonance and excess nasal air emission, (2) hoarse/breathy phonation with an overlay of wet-gurgly quality and limited pitch and loudness variation, and (3) imprecise articulation, particularly on high-pressure consonants. Moderate weakness of the velopharyngeal musculature on the left was evident on examination of the oral cavity. Acoustic and speech aerodynamic studies showed reduced maximum phonation time, a fundamental frequency of 200 Hz, aberrant phonatory jitter and shimmer, and increased glottic airflow. Videostroboscopic laryngeal examination showed (1) profound pooling of saliva in the laryngeal vestibule and pyriform sinuses, (2) intermittent aspiration of secretions, (3) unilateral adductor vocal fold paralysis on the left with the fold positioned in the near-abducted position at rest, (4) persistent wide glottal chink at the mid-line during phonatory efforts, and (5) failure of the involved vocal fold to alter length and tension during attempts at pitch and loudness variations.

Because of concerns about the patient's potential for aspiration and swallowing dysfunction, a videofluorographic study of swallow was ordered. Results showed significant aspiration and nasopharyngeal reflux on all consistencies from weakness of the pharyngeal musculature and delayed pharyngeal-swallow reflex, poor elevation of the larynx and velopharynx, and incompetent glottal closure.

Worksheet

Salient symptoms/signs	Test results	Impressions

This worksheet is to be used for recording relevant diagnostic observations. The blank illustration is to be used for identifying and sketching the suspected site of lesion(s). These steps should be completed prior to turning to the Impressions and illustrated site of lesion.

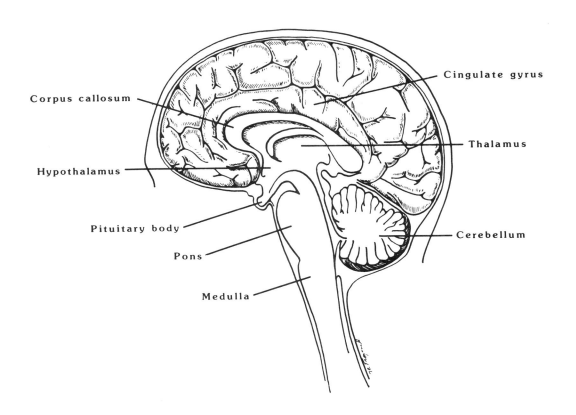

Corpus callosum

Cingulate gyrus

Hypothalamus

Thalamus

Pituitary body

Pons

Cerebellum

Medulla

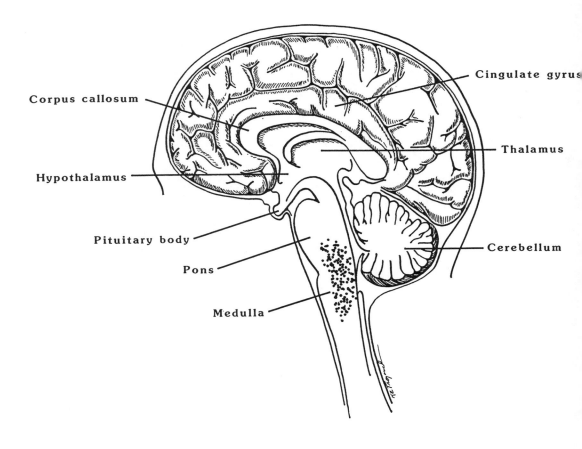

Corpus callosum

Cingulate gyrus

Hypothalamus

Thalamus

Pituitary body

Pons

Cerebellum

Medulla

Impressions Flaccid dysarthria involving the laryngeal and velopharyngeal musculature; dysphagia, from Xth nerve damage on the left; pontomedullary
involvement.

Discussion In this patient, damage to the left Vagus nerve was evident from the
flaccid laryngeal and velopharyngeal symptoms and signs. The site of
lesion was believed to be at the brainstem level (intracranial), implicating the palatopharyngeal plexus as well as the superior and recurrent
laryngeal nerve distributions. When a vocal fold is paralyzed in the fully
abducted position and there is co-occurring ipsilateral pharyngeal involvement, a high vagal nerve lesion (either intra-axial or extra-axial)
is expected. The co-occurring dysphagia in this patient's case would
suggest more widespread brainstem involvement, including impairment
of the pontomedullary reflexive "swallowing center."

For this patient, the findings were substantiated by perceptual, acoustic, and laryngeal stroboscopic analyses as well as videofluorographic
study of swallow. The patient underwent a thyroplastic procedure for
medialization of the left vocal fold. Postoperatively, he continued to
have a mildly hoarse-breathy voice, with limited pitch and loudness
range. However, maximum phonation time increased, fundamental
frequency decreased to a more natural 135 Hz, jitter and shimmer fell
to within normal limits, and harmonic/noise ratio and laryngeal resistance measures were moderately improved.

For the velopharyngeal dysfunction, a palatal lift was adapted to the
patient's existing upper denture. Hypernasal resonance was mildly
improved and airflow/air pressure dynamics showed marginal gains.

Swallowing therapy initially implemented thickened liquids, progressing to soft and semisolid, with no evidence of aspiration. At the time
of this report, he was tolerating a general diet without difficulty.

Voice therapy has stressed improvement of vocal quality and loudness controls, whereas pitch control may be difficult to achieve inasmuch as the thyroplastic procedure does not directly influence functions of the cricothyroid musculature, which chiefly regulates pitch.

69-Year-Old Male with History of Coronary Artery Disease and Carcinoma Has Change in Speech

History   This 69-year-old male was referred to speech pathology by his internist for evaluation of a change in voice following colostomy two years prior to examination. His prior medical history was rather vast, being most significant both for coronary artery disease with congestive heart failure, and for sigmoid colostomy for rectal carcinoma, of which he was free at last examination. Current medications included amoxapine (Asendin), 50 mg 4 times daily; digoxin (Digoxin), 2 mg daily; hydralazine hydrochloride (Hydralazine), 50 mg twice daily; and furosemide (Lasix), 40 mg 3 times daily.

Examination   Laryngologic examination was within normal limits. There was no history of dysphagia, dyspnea, or nasal reflux. Voice was moderately-severely wet-hoarse in quality, monopitched, and judged louder than normal. The patient did admit to being depressed secondary to the recent loss of his wife, and had also noted a progressive deterioration in the legibility of his handwriting.

Examination of the motor speech mechanism was significant for mildly masked facies with a palmomental reflex elicited to the left. Glabellar tap was negative. The tongue protruded symmetrically to the midline and laterally, without compromise in strength. The velopharynx was symmetrical at rest and during phonation. A gag reflex was elicited. With the exception of an edentulous mouth managed by dentures, the remainder of the examination was within normal limits.

Oral diadochokinetic and sequential articulatory motion rates were mildly irregular and decreased in amplitude, while articulation in connected speech was marked by variable articulatory breakdown, secondary to sound distortion and omission. Speaking rate was marked by an increased rate in segments with short rushes of speech. Respiratory support for speech and resonation were considered within normal limits. There were no language findings, although a sample of handwriting suggested micrographia.

Gross walking movements were bradykinetic. There was no limb rigidity with reinforcement, although moderate rigidity of the head and neck with reinforcement was evident. Gaze in every direction was normal. Finger-to-nose testing and extension of the limbs suggested fine physiologic tremor. There was no resting tremor.

Salient symptoms/signs	Test results	Impressions

This worksheet is to be used for recording relevant diagnostic observations. The blank illustration is to be used for identifying and sketching the suspected site of lesion(s). These steps should be completed prior to turning to the Impressions and illustrated site of lesion.

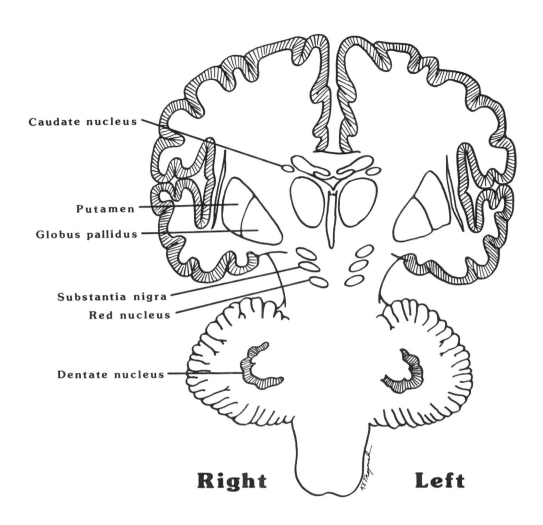

Caudate nucleus

Putamen

Globus pallidus

Substantia nigra

Red nucleus

Dentate nucleus

Right   **Left**

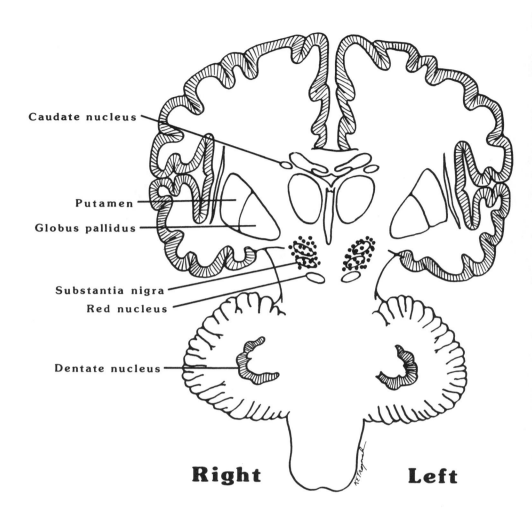

Caudate nucleus

Putamen

Globus pallidus

Substantia nigra

Red nucleus

Dentate nucleus

Right **Left**

Impressions Hypokinetic (parkinsonian) dysarthria.

Discussion The primary extrapyramidal features, including dysarthria, bradykinesia, and rigidity, were judged pathognomonic of parkinsonism. Reviewing the various drugs he had been taking, we discovered that amoxapine (Asendin) may have induced the parkinsonian symptoms. The medication was temporarily discontinued to determine if it indeed was the offending agent. One month following initial examination and discontinuation of the drug, substantial improvements in the patient's voice and motor speech skills were evident. He continued, however, to have periods of depression.

Although amoxapine is not considered a dopamine inhibitor, conceivably in this patient it adversely affected the cholinergic-dopaminergic balance. This may have created "tardive" parkinsonian sequelae. Usually, tardive dyskinesias are induced by overdoses of drugs within the "thiazine" group. Significant extrapyramidal signs are infrequent side effects of amoxapine. The dysarthrias that result from such side effects generally fall under the hyperkinetic category. In this case, however, the side effects of amoxapine were hypokinetic in nature, marked by a paucity rather than an increase in movement. Along with improvement in motor speech signs following discontinuation of the drug, the patient's handwriting improved substantially and was no longer considered micrographic.

9-Year-Old Male with History of Influenza and Lethargy Has Language Disturbance

History   The patient had followed a normal developmental history until age 9, when he experienced moderate to severe episodes of influenza and mild pneumonia. He was admitted to hospital and routine treatments were instituted. Five days after admission, he began vomiting relentlessly and was lethargic and unusually tired. Two days later he exhibited signs of disorientation, delirium, combativeness, and hyperventilation.

Liver scans and EEG were abnormal, the latter primarily focal over the left temporal lobe. Three days later he experienced generalized seizures that were not adequately controlled by medication. Late that evening, he sank into a deep coma marked by decerebrate rigidity; loss of oculocephalic and deep tendon reflexes; large, fixed pupils; and respiratory arrest. EEG revealed diffuse arrhythmic delta activity. The patient remained comatose for approximately three weeks, followed by gradual awakening.

Examination   On initial examination, the patient was moderately alert and responsive. He did, however, have difficulty following simple one-step verbal commands. Contextual speech was fluent, lengthy, and generally grammatical; however, there was a lack of semantic relationship between answers and stimulus questions. Naming was variably accurate. He inconsistently recognized isolated letters and could read some simple words but not phrases or sentences. He could copy shapes and write some simple words, but not sentences to dictation. Knowledge of orientation was equivocal due to the communicative impairment. There were no motor speech findings.

CT scan revealed marked prominence of the left lateral ventricles and generalized cerebral edema on the left side. Repeat liver scans showed diffuse steatosis (fatty degeneration) with mild inflammatory changes. EEG remained abnormal with focal signs over the midposterior left hemisphere. Mild but persistent truncal ataxia and spastic quadriparesis were detected, as were associated bilateral Babinski signs. Sensory function was normal.

Salient symptoms/signs	Test results	Impressions

This worksheet is to be used for recording relevant diagnostic observations. The blank illustration is to be used for identifying and sketching the suspected site of lesion(s). These steps should be completed prior to turning to the Impressions and illustrated site of lesion.

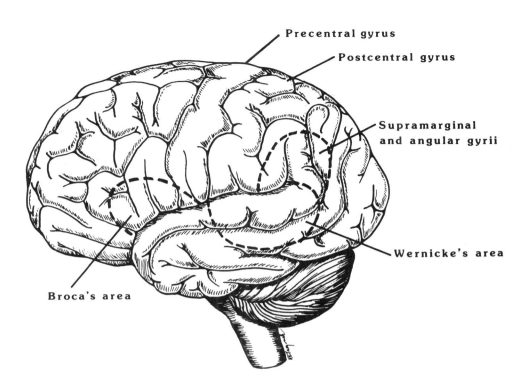

Precentral gyrus

Postcentral gyrus

Supramarginal
and angular gyrii

Wernicke's area

Broca's area

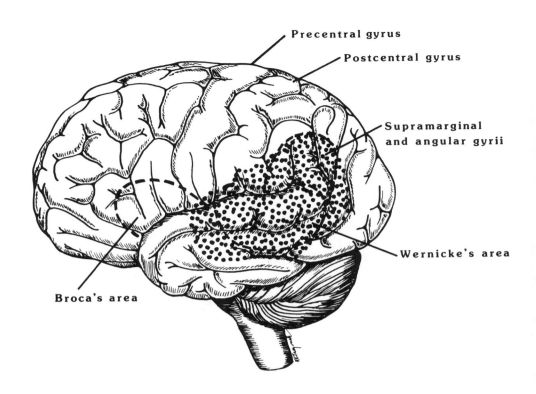

Precentral gyrus

Postcentral gyrus

Supramarginal
and angular gyrii

Wernicke's area

Broca's area

Impressions   Aphasia due to Reye's syndrome.

Discussion   Reye's syndrome, first described in 1963, is a disease that typically affects individuals between the ages of 1 and 23, the average age of onset being 8 years. Males are afflicted more frequently than females, and over 90 percent of cases are Caucasian. The mortality rate is approximately 40 percent, and 11 percent of those who survive have various neurologic symptoms.

The cause of the syndrome is not completely understood. It tends to occur soon after the child recovers from an episode of upper respiratory infection such as Type B influenza or chicken pox.

Reye's syndrome may progress through five stages. In stage one, relentless vomiting, lethargy, and sleepiness occur. In stages two and three, disorientation, delirium, combativeness, hyperventilation, liver dysfunction, and abnormal EEG patterns are observed. Stage four is characterized by decerebrate rigidity, cerebral edema, and deepening coma. In stage five, seizures, loss of deep tendon reflexes, respiratory arrests, and abnormal EEG patterns prevail.

The diagnosis of Reye's syndrome is usually withheld until late in stage two or early in stage three. Our patient progressed through the five stages of this disease within two weeks after he suffered from the flu and pneumonia. The diagnosis of Reye's syndrome was considered soon after the episodes of violent vomiting, behavioral changes, and liver dysfunction.

The language deficits exhibited by our patient were felt to be consistent with aphasia, although his knowledge of orientation, abstract thought, and reasoning skills could not be adequately assessed. The ataxia and spasticity were suggestive of cerebellum and corticospinal tract involvement, respectively.

Mannitol and dexamethasone (Decadron) were prescribed to reduce cerebral swelling. Speech-language therapy was initiated, with emphasis on auditory comprehension and expressive language skills. Improvement was minimal over the course of six months, due in part to recurring episodes of upper respiratory infections.

21-Year-Old Male with Clos and Speech Disturbance

History Although he had sustained multiple injurie:
the forehead, right mandible, zygomatic ar(
21-year-old male college student was alert,
admission to emergency room following a motor vehicle accident. The
superficial injuries were treated successfully by the attending physician,
who also noted labored, periodically inarticulate, and breathy speech
in the presence of apparent normal language.

Skull x-rays, CT scans, and angiography were normal. Because of
difficulty handling his own secretions and a weak cough, he underwent
a laryngologic examination that revealed essentially fixed vocal cords
in the abducted position with only a trace of approximation on request
for voice. An emergency tracheostomy was performed and the patient
transferred to the intensive care unit.

Examination Examination revealed: (1) right facial paresis marked by difficulty with
forehead wrinkling, winking of the eye, and retracting the corner of
the mouth; (2) mildly irregular bilabial alternate motion rates, with
impaired labial consonant production in words and contexts; (3) a
decreased gag reflex and associated bilateral velopharyngeal paralysis
and hypernasality and nasal air emission; (4) aphonia secondary to
tracheostomy, although when the tube was occluded voice was severely breathy and hoarse; (5) paresis of the tongue on the left with
associated deviation to that side on protrusion; (6) mild-moderate
impaired lingual alternate motion rates with associated decreased range
and control of movement; and (7) impaired articulation in words and
context.

The results of facial and lingual electromyography (EMG) were equivocal. The patient underwent surgery to reposition the arytenoid car-
tilages to enhance vocal cord approximation. He was discharged from
hospital six weeks later. Prior to discharge, the tracheostomy was
closed. He failed to keep routine follow-up appointments.

Eighteen months following the injury he sought further evaluation.
Examination now revealed atrophic changes involving the right side of
the face, left side of the tongue, and portions of the velopharynx. The
vocal cords were bowed on phonation but approximated the midline.
The patient's speech was characterized by continuous, severe hypernasality with nasal air emission, hoarseness and breathiness, and impaired articulation marked by distortion of consonant sounds. The
patient did not complain of difficulty swallowing.

Worksheet

Salient symptoms/signs	Test results	Impressions

This worksheet is to be used for recording relevant diagnostic observations. The blank illustration is to be used for identifying and sketching the suspected site of lesion(s). These steps should be completed prior to turning to the Impressions and illustrated site of lesion.

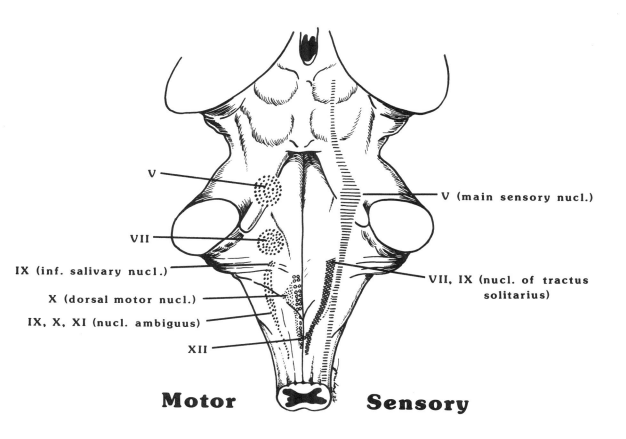

V

V (main sensory nucl.)

VII

IX (inf. salivary nucl.)

X (dorsal motor nucl.)

IX, X, XI (nucl. ambiguus)

XII

VII, IX (nucl. of tractus
solitarius)

Motor   **Sensory**

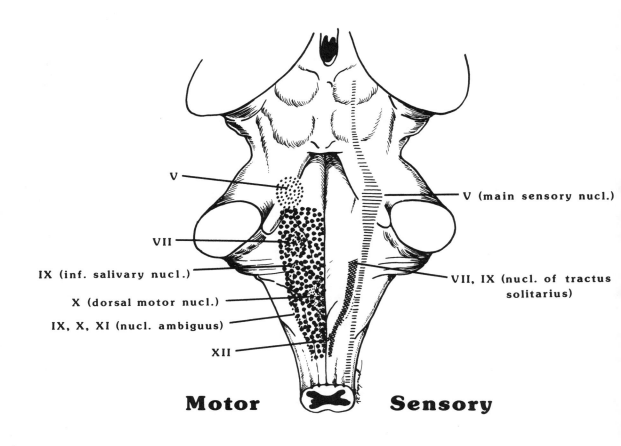

Motor   **Sensory**

V

V (main sensory nucl.)

VII

IX (inf. salivary nucl.)

X (dorsal motor nucl.)

IX, X, XI (nucl. ambiguus)

XII

VII, IX (nucl. of tractus solitarius)

Impressions   Flaccid dysarthria secondary to polyneuropathy of traumatic origin.

Discussion   Atrophy and fasciculations, cardinal signs of lower motor neuron impairment, may not be clinically observable or detectable until several weeks or months after the insult. Our patient suffered multiple cranial nerve involvement resulting in flaccid dysarthria, manifested initially by paresis of musculature and concurrent impaired resonation, phonation, and articulation. The bilateral velopharyngeal and laryngeal signs pointed to involvement at the level of the lower brainstem, although this could not be confirmed radiographically.

There is an important clinical distinction between a peripheral facial paralysis, as in our patient, and the central facial paresis that occurs with pyramidal tract (supranuclear) lesions. In the former, the entire face may be involved on the side affected, including the musculature that wrinkles the forehead and aids in closing the eyelid. Auditory acuity may be depressed because of co-occurring involvement of the stapedius muscle in the middle ear. In the latter, the lower two-thirds of the opposite side of the face is involved, but the forehead, eyelid, and auditory functions are preserved. Atrophy and fasciculations do not occur in central facial paresis.

In our patient, the patent velopharynx and larynx with resultant continuous resonatory and phonatory signs are consistent with IXth and Xth cranial nerve involvement at or above (extracranial or intracranial) the inferior ganglia. When the pyramidal tract is involved, however, the speech signs may be variable and consistent with spastic dysarthria.

Usually unilateral peripheral or central paresis of the tongue gives rise to only minimal articulation difficulties. In our patient, however, articulation was significantly affected because of co-occurring resonatory and phonatory impairment.

To improve his resonance, our patient was fitted with a palatal lift. This device, along with laryngeal surgery and speech therapy, provided a good prognosis for improving speech intelligibility. However, he withdrew from therapy and did not keep follow-up appointments.

84-Year-Old Female with Right Side Weakness and Unintelligible Speech

History   The patient is an 84-year-old moderately hypertensive female nursing home resident who fell to the floor on the day of admission. The nursing staff noted that she was having difficulty speaking and that the right side of her face drooped. Further, she did not use her preferred right arm and appeared to favor her left leg.

Examination   Medical history from the patient was impossible in that her verbal expression was unintelligible. She appeared to understand all instructions and readily followed nonverbal commands. Her pupils were equal and reacted normally to light. The lower two-thirds of her face on the right side was paretic; she drooled from that side. The tongue protruded symmetrically to the midline, without compromise in strength. The soft palate was symmetrical at rest and during attempts at phonation. A normal gag reflex was elicited.

The patient adequately handled her own secretions; she did not complain of difficulty swallowing. Heart and lungs were normal; blood pressure was 160/90. The right upper and lower extremities were moderately weak; some pronator drift was noted on the right upper extremity. A Babinski sign was elicited on the right; deep tendon reflexes were reactive and equal. The patient was admitted to hospital for further evaluation. Admitting CT scan and EEG were normal.

On speech pathology examination, the patient was notably frustrated concerning her communication deficit. Articulatory diadochokinetic and sequential motion rates were grossly irregular. Of isolated vowels to be imitated, 69 percent were distorted. Articulation in conversational speech was generally unintelligible and marked by variable sound addition, omission, substitution, and transposition errors.

Further, voice-voiceless transpositions such as /t/ for /d/, were noted. Errors appeared to be rendered as a function of speech complexity; that is, articulatory precision breaking down beyond one or two syllables. Articulatory groping was evident. A test of oral praxis was marked by 57 percent error. Utterances were short and rate variable, both probably compensatory strategies for the articulatory imprecision. Phonation, resonation, and respiration were within normal limits.

Assessment of language function revealed normal auditory comprehension of simple to complex commands. Assessment of auditory retention by means of a verbal response was difficult because of the motor speech deficit. However, she was able to write a response with the nonpreferred left upper extremity. Auditory retention for digits was 5, and for syllables and words, 15 and 12, respectively. She missed none of the items used to assess mental computation. Again, for paper-pencil calculation, she used the left upper extremity. No errors were rendered for this portion of the examination. She was able to copy simple geometric forms and write, albeit poorly orthographically, with the right upper extremity.

Salient symptoms/signs	Test results	Impressions

This worksheet is to be used for recording relevant diagnostic observations. The blank illustration is to be used for identifying and sketching the suspected site of lesion(s). These steps should be completed prior to turning to the Impressions and illustrated site of lesion.

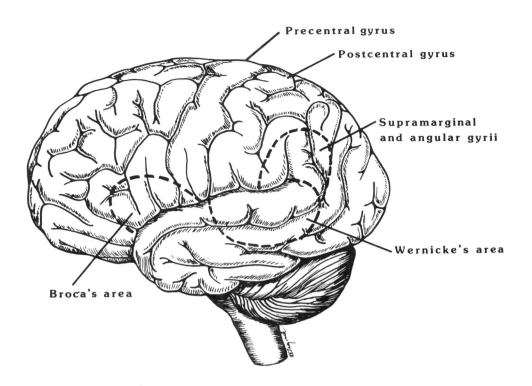

Precentral gyrus

Postcentral gyrus

Supramarginal
and angular gyrii

Wernicke's area

Broca's area

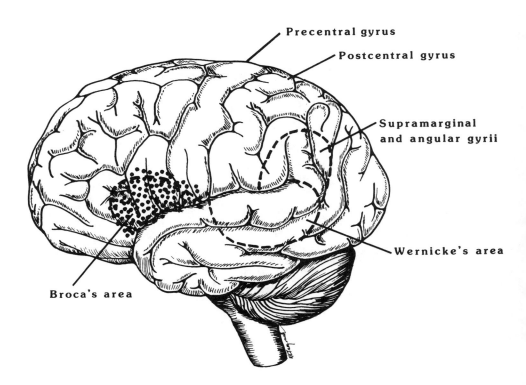

Impressions   Speech/oral apraxia due to involvement of the left lateral-inferior frontal lobe.

Discussion   This patient's right extremity and lower two-thirds facial signs are consistent with involvement of the left pyramidal tract, most likely secondary to an embolic infarct. The dysarthria that may result from such involvement is usually transient and mild. It may, however, prove significant in pure motor or capsular infarcts that impair lingual function as well.

A lesion of the left frontal lobe may involve the pyramidal pathway and motor speech programming area as well. Apraxia of speech and frequently oral apraxia more often than not co-occur with aphasia. In such situations the task for the examiner is to differentiate between those signs that are motor programming from those that are language processing in nature.

The diagnostic features of apraxia of speech—which include articulatory imprecision secondary to sound omission, addition, transposition, and articulatory groping—are some of the cardinal signs that help differentiate apraxic from aphasic errors. Further, the prosodic and rate problems that also occur in apraxia may be compensatory for either the articulatory imprecision or components of the apraxia itself.

History   The patient is a 25-year-old female involved in an automobile accident. At the accident site, she was unresponsive but breathing on her own. Her pupils were unequal and unreactive. Her blood pressure was normal. In route to the hospital, she developed decerebrate posturing and her breathing became labored. On admission, she was intubated and hyperventilated. Skull and cervical spine films proved negative for fractures; chest x-ray was normal. Head CT scan revealed (1) a shearing tear of the corpus callosum and (2) multiple and diffuse focal hemorrhagic contusions. For brain swelling, she was started on prophylactic dexamethasone (Decadron) and Mannitol. A deep left cheek laceration was cleaned and sutured. Her pupils had become equal and reactive; the corneal reflexes were intact bilaterally. Her tendon reflexes were equal and symmetrical, and she withdrew from painful stimuli. Bilateral Babinski signs were elicited. Her Glasgow coma score was six (severe coma).

On the day following admission, the patient was taken to the operating room for placement of an intracranial pressure monitor. The ventriculostomy was taken down two days later and the patient was extubated and weaned from the ventilator. Her intracranial pressure remained low; her coma score stayed at six.

Over the course of the next two weeks, the patient became more alert and responsive, could initiate conversation and move her limbs. She was transferred to the rehabilitation unit for comprehensive evaluation and treatment.

Examination   Neuromotor examination showed (1) ataxia necessitating assistance with virtually all motor tasks, (2) decreased aerobic capacity and endurance, and (3) reduced psychomotor speed and strength in all limbs. Range of motion for all extremities was within normal limits. All reflexes were equal and normal bilaterally.

Neurolinguistic evaluation revealed (1) markedly impaired auditory-verbal memory, (2) sustained attention deficits, (3) word retrieval and fluency difficulties, (4) verbal abstract reasoning impairment, (5) severe memory disturbances (involving all areas—immediate, recent, and remote), and (6) emotional lability.

Motor speech examination showed (1) resting tremor at approximately 5 Hz involving the velopharyngeal and laryngeal musculature as documented by clinical electroglottographic and endoscopic analyses; (2) maximum phonation time of less than eight seconds; (3) increased glottal air flow and decreased resistance with values of 375 cc/sec, and 15 cmH20/lit/sec, respectively; (4) aberrant vocal jitter and shimmer (pitch perturbation and intensity variation, respectively); and (5) vocal tremor, intermittent breathiness, and variable hypernasal resonance most notable during vowel prolongation and production of short sentences and conversational speech samples. Other motor speech findings were of lesser significance.

463

Salient symptoms/signs	Test results	Impressions

This worksheet is to be used for recording relevant diagnostic observations. The blank illustration is to be used for identifying and sketching the suspected site of lesion(s). These steps should be completed prior to turning to the Impressions and illustrated site of lesion.

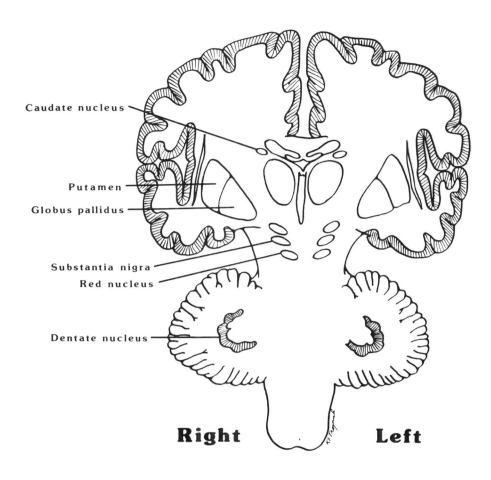

Caudate nucleus

Putamen

Globus pallidus

Substantia nigra
Red nucleus

Dentate nucleus

Right　　　　**Left**

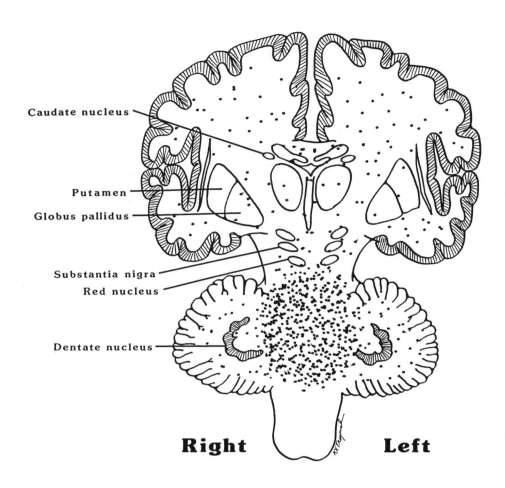

Caudate nucleus

Putamen

Globus pallidus

Substantia nigra
Red nucleus

Dentate nucleus

Right   **Left**

Impressions   Generalized intellectual impairment, hyperkinetic dysarthria (quick form) manifested by palatal pharyngeal laryngeal myoclonus status post closed head injury with diffuse axonal shear.

Discussion   Comprehensive treatment focused on improving balance, posturing, speed of psychomotor response, abstract reasoning skills, attention span and memory, word fluency, and sequential thought processes. Speech therapy per se was not indicated for the dysarthria. Palatal pharyngeal laryngeal myoclonus is thought to be due to involvement of the Guillane-Molaret triangle (dentato-rubro-olivary tracts of the brainstem). Aberrant contractions of the bulbar musculature generally between 2 and 4 Hz are most evident at rest. On vowel prolongation, regular changes in volume are perceptible and can be identified instrumentally. In some cases, as in this patient, myoclonus can be subtle and may go unrecognized—stressing the importance of careful examination of the oral speech mechanism both at rest and during speech. Unfortunately, palatal pharyngeal laryngeal myoclonus is often resistent to pharmacologic therapy. There are, however, some reports of the efficacy of trihexyphenidyl (Artane) and 5 Hydroxytryptophan (5HTP) being effective for reducing movements in some patients.

64-Year-Old Male with History of Myocardial Infarction Has Nausea, Diplopia, Vertigo, and Speech Disturbance

History   This patient is a 64-year-old male with a history of hypertension, heavy smoking, and myocardial infarction. On the day of admission, he awoke to find himself on the floor. On arising, he was dizzy and his speech slurred. He was unable to walk or stand by himself. In the emergency room, he exhibited nausea, intermittent diplopia, vertigo, and slurred speech.

Examination   Bilateral rotary nystagmus was noted. The right side of his body revealed reduced response to pinprick and light touch testing. Cerebellar findings were normal. CT scan with and without contrast, including routine cuts of the posterior fossa, were within normal limits.

Hiccuping at rest, occurring at a frequency of approximately 3 to 4 Hz, was evident. The right side of the face appeared mildly asymmetrical with depression of the nasolabial fold and flattening of the orbicularis oculi and frontalis muscles on that side; lip seal and strength were normal.

Examination of the velopharyngeal mechanism suggested mild velar asymmetry with depression on the right at rest; during vowel prolongation the velum pulled to the left. At rest, quick posterior-superior movements of the velum were noted in synchrony with audible hiccuping. Tongue protrusion was mildly asymmetrical, deviating to the right without compromise in strength or range of movement.

Oral diadochokinetic rates were slow and moderately irregular, while sequential motion rates were mildly irregular but rendered at a normal rate. During connected speech, there was variable articulatory breakdown with distortions of consonant sounds. On occasion, there was repetition of individual phonemes. Articulatory intelligibility was moderately disturbed.

Voice quality was harsh as well as wet-hoarse and intermittently breathy. On prolongation of a neutral vowel, there were instances of variable pitch as well as downward pitch breaks. Again, instances of hiccuping were noted. Indirect rigid fiberoptic laryngoscopy suggested incomplete vocal cord approximation because of right vocal cord paresis. The patient also noted that he occasionally choked on liquids and his own saliva.

Speaking rate was fast with increased rate in segments. The patient felt that his speaking rate had indeed increased since hospitalization. Both respiration and resonation appeared within normal limits for speech.

Salient symptoms/signs	Test results	Impressions

This worksheet is to be used for recording relevant diagnostic observations. The blank illustration is to be used for identifying and sketching the suspected site of lesion(s). These steps should be completed prior to turning to the Impressions and illustrated site of lesion.

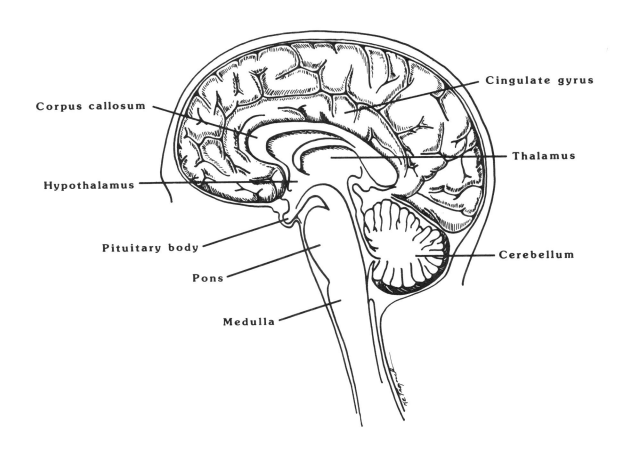

Corpus callosum

Cingulate gyrus

Hypothalamus

Thalamus

Pituitary body

Pons

Cerebellum

Medulla

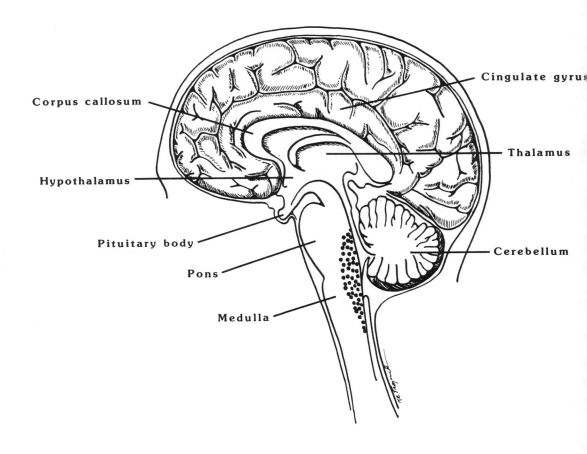

Corpus callosum

Cingulate gyrus

Thalamus

Hypothalamus

Pituitary body

Cerebellum

Pons

Medulla

64-Year-Old Male with History of Myocardial Infarction Has Nausea, Diplopia, Vertigo, and Speech Disturbance

Impressions   Mixed hyperkinetic (quick)-flaccid dysarthria.

Discussion   In part, many of the findings for this patient were consistent with *Wallenberg's syndrome,* caused by an infarct in the zone supplied by the posterior inferior cerebellar artery. Typically it is characterized by dysarthria, dysphagia; ipsilateral decrease in pain, temperature, and sensation of the face; and contralateral loss of pain and temperature sensation of the trunk and extremities. The left sensory deficit was difficult to confirm in this patient, although the hypesthesia of both the right arm and leg was evident. There was no decrease in pain or temperature, however. The bilateral rotary nystagmus was consistent with brainstem involvement.

The nucleus ambiguus, either unilaterally or bilaterally, can be affected in Wallenberg's syndrome. This patient's motor speech symptoms and signs appeared to be unilateral. His right facial, velopharyngeal, lingual, and laryngeal musculature paresis were suggestive of unilateral involvement of the VIIth, IXth, Xth, and XIIth cranial nerves on that side while the hiccuping, vocal harshness, and increased speaking rate were considered signs of hyperkinesia.

Hiccups, which may be a form of myoclonus, are an interesting clinical sign and may arise from a number of different causes, including irritation of the phrenic nerve or vascular or neoplastic changes involving the brain stem. In this patient's case, it was felt that the etiology was related to a probable brainstem stroke with involvement of the striatal-pallidal tracts. Valproic acid may be of benefit in treating intractible hiccups.

At the time of discharge, the patient was able to dress himself and was generally able to walk independently. Although the dysarthria persisted, he no longer had instances of dysphagia on liquids or saliva and the hiccuping had resolved. Interestingly, the latter had not been treated medically during hospitalization.

51-Year-Old Female with History of Heart Disease Has a Change in Language

History   The patient is a 51-year-old female whose prior medical history was significant for hypertension and mitral valve stenosis, both of which had been managed medically. On the morning of admission to the emergency room, she awoke with garbled speech. On transfer to the hospital, she was lethargic but arousable.

Examination   The patient was lethargic but arousable on examination. Reflexes of the right limbs were hyperactive with associated hypertonicity and weakness. There was a question of decreased sensation on the right. Emergency CT scan was normal; EEG revealed left hemispheric slowing. The patient was able to handle her own secretions and take liquids and solids. She was not in respiratory distress; heart rhythms were acceptable for her.

Examination of the motor speech mechanism revealed a question of mild right central facial paresis. The Vth, IXth, Xth, XIth, and XIIth cranial nerves were clinically within normal limits. When alert, she was able to complete the majority of oral and speech praxis tasks without error. Visual fields appeared normal.

Assessment of language function revealed that 30 percent of the items requiring knowledge of one-step commands, 80 percent of the items requiring understanding of right-left orientation, and 90 percent of the items requiring comprehension of two-step commands were missed. She was unable to retain more than 4 digits forward or sentences beyond 9 words. With prompting, she was able to match 70 percent of common objects and pictures of common objects and to recognize and label 50 percent of isolated letters.

Forty percent of the items requiring recognition and comprehension of isolated words, and 80 percent of the items requiring comprehension of simple-to-complex sentences were missed. Of the items requiring a verbal label for common objects and pictures of common objects, 60 percent were missed. She also missed 60 percent of the items used to assess mental computation skills, and 50 percent of the items used to measure paper-pencil calculation performance. Of the items to be written to dictation, including letters, words, and sentences, 80 percent were missed.

Conversational speech was notably perseverative and neologistic. Frequently her response to stimuli was, "Well, I know that; well, I know that." Although she was variably able to express her needs through gesture and verbalization, she was unable to use writing for expression.

Salient symptoms/signs	Test results	Impressions

This worksheet is to be used for recording relevant diagnostic observations. The blank illustration is to be used for identifying and sketching the suspected site of lesion(s). These steps should be completed prior to turning to the Impressions and illustrated site of lesion.

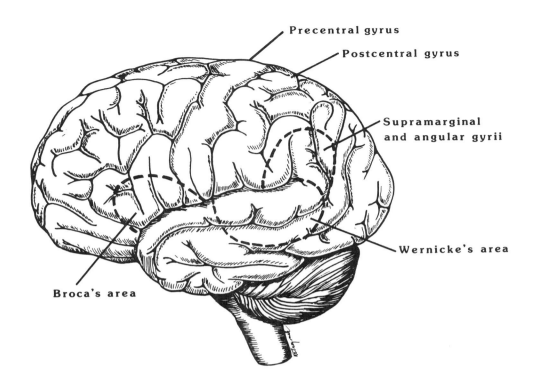

Precentral gyrus

Postcentral gyrus

Supramarginal
and angular gyrii

Wernicke's area

Broca's area

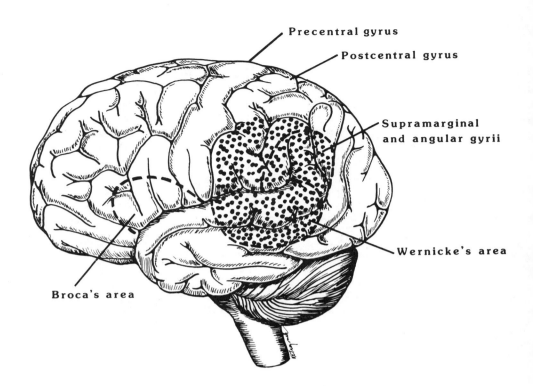

Impressions   Aphasia following left hemisphere stroke, possibly embolic in origin.

Discussion   Although not confirmed, the history of heart disease would suggest that the patient's stroke was secondary to a thromboembolic event, possibly originating in the heart or cardiac vessels.

The patient's right body and central facial symptoms implicate the left pyramidal system. Her decreased sensation may have been secondary to periSylvian or periRolandic involvement not an infrequent finding when the postcentral gyrus, the primary central connection for pain and temperature proprioception and touch, is disturbed.

The language findings are fairly typical for aphasia crossing all language modalities. In this instance decoding and encoding are deficient and characterized by perseveration and neologistic distortion.

In neologistic distortions, frequently there is a semantic relationship between the target stimulus and the response rendered by a patient. For example, in an attempt to elicit a label for the word "pen" following object presentation, the patient offers "preen." With the exception of the intrusive /r/ and prolongation of the vowel /e/, the response is accurate. Similar findings hold true for dysnomic errors as well, in which a patient may label a "shirt" a "jacket."

Our patient was placed on anticoagulants and seen for speech therapy directed primarily toward auditory and visual comprehension. She was also being evaluated for mitral valve replacement. At the time of discharge from the hospital, the patient remained dysphasic, although improvement had been made in all areas of language function. The motor and sensory signs had virtually resolved.

20-Year-Old Male with Traumatic Injuries

History   The patient is a 20-year-old, right-handed male college student who was in good health before involvement in a motor vehicle accident. On emergency room arrival he was in deep coma and had decorticate posturing with spasticity, greater on the right. His pelvis and right clavicle were fractured. After intubation and being placed on a ventilator, his pupils became more reactive. Multiple abrasions and contusions of the head were noted, most pronounced in the right temporal bone area; blood was found in the right ear canal.

Serum electrolyte, blood culture, and urine samples proved negative; an increased white blood cell count and dropping hematocrit were discovered. CT scan of the head demonstrated interventricular bleeding with acute blood in the lateral ventricles and scattered hemorrhagic areas in both the right and left frontal lobes. EEG indicated diffuse dysrhythmic slowing without epileptiform activity, more pronounced on the right side.

The bony and superficial wounds were treated and the patient was transferred to the ICU. He was placed on intravenous Mannitol and dexamethasone (Decadron) and dehydrated to control cerebral edema.

By the fifth day following admission, the patient opened his eyes widely to painful stimuli, was decorticate on the left, decerebrate on the right, and spastic in all extremities. By the 12th day, he demonstrated coma vigilance: eyes wide open, no response to auditory or visual stimulation, and decorticate flexion and spasticity, bilaterally.

Repeat CT scans during this time revealed gradual absorption and healing of the contusions and hemorrhages in the ventricular system, along with the accumulation of low density extraocular fluid in the left frontal lobe region, compatible with a small subdural hygroma (sac or cyst filled with fluid). By the 28th day, postinjury, he was awake, could occasionally lift a finger on command, and eat some food by mouth. At that time, he was transferred to the rehabilitation unit, where he underwent comprehensive evaluation and treatment for the next several months.

Examination   The following summarizes test results at 14 months postinjury:

Neuromotor examination revealed (1) slowed gait, with moderate flexion hypertonicity and weakness of the right hip and upper and lower extremities, (2) mild shoulder flexion on the left, (3) moderate dysdiadochokinesia of both upper and lower extremities on the right, and (4) moderately brisk deep tendon reflexes bilaterally.

Neuropsychologic evaluation showed impairment in the areas of spatial orientation, reaction time, judgment, and short-term memory, rated moderate to severe in degree. He also had signs of denial, was clinically depressed and prone to reactive physical tantrum.

The patient was nonverbal; he used a portable communication device to type his responses and to make his wishes known. Profound short-term memory deficits affected auditory and visual retention. "Written" (typed) expressions were only mildly distorted for vocabulary, syntax, and meaning. The patient was known to write short stories and poetry between treatment sessions.

Motor speech examination identified (1) mild to moderate unilateral right side paresis, hypertonicity, and discoordination of the orofacial musculature; (2) verbal efforts characterized by high-pitched squeals, intermittent but frequent periods of whispered or no phonation, loudness outbursts; (3) intact involuntary vocalizations including coughing and throat clearing (laryngologic examination was normal); (4) profoundly impaired articulation rendering his speech attempts unintelligible; and (5) visible struggle to posture the articulators correctly.

Worksheet

Salient symptoms/signs	Test results	Impressions

This worksheet is to be used for recording relevant diagnostic observations. The blank illustration is to be used for identifying and sketching the suspected site of lesion(s). These steps should be completed prior to turning to the Impressions and illustrated site of lesion.

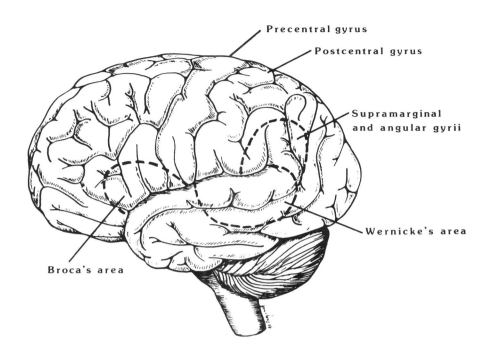

Precentral gyrus

Postcentral gyrus

Supramarginal
and angular gyrii

Wernicke's area

Broca's area

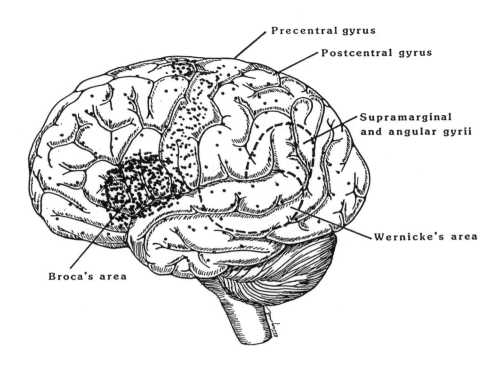

Precentral gyrus

Postcentral gyrus

Supramarginal
and angular gyrii

Wernicke's area

Broca's area

Impressions   Dyspraxia of speech (including dyspraxia of phonation)/oral dyspraxia complex; generalized intellectual impairment associated with severe closed head injury.

Discussion   The patient's spastic hemiplegia on the right and unilateral orofacial pathophysiologic features were suggestive of involvement of the left corticospinal and corticobulbar tracts (pyramidal system). Although left side difficulties were only mild in degree, they implicated the right corticospinal tract as well. CT data supported clinical findings, showing bifrontal-hemispheric involvement as well. It was felt that the patient's severe motor speech planning disorder (dyspraxia of speech plus phonation) was associated with involvement of the left cerebral hemisphere areas 44 and 45 as well as the supplemental motor cortex. He was not only unable to access or volitionally program muscular movements for articulation, but also the laryngeal mechanism for voice. These findings, in the absence of comparable neuromuscular involvement, further supported the diagnosis of a motor speech planning disorder.

Abnormal motor speech planning characteristics of articulatory groping, struggle, discoordinated efforts to initiate speech (and voice!) are tantamount to differential diagnosis of dyspraxia of speech. In our patient, the phonatory component was so severe and interruptive that it confused differential diagnosis initially. Moreover, the nature of the phonatory component did not become clear until the patient successfully completed a treatment plan that focused on phonation.

Believing that the patient would not benefit from articulatory-prosodic exercises until he gained control of phonation, treatment initially focused on improving voice motor control using a metronome as a pacing device. He was also receiving physical, occupational, and neurocognitive therapy. Approximately three years after his closed head injury, the patient was discharged from all treatment programs with intelligible speech and mild right hemiplegia. He was living independently with minimal supervision, able to jog on his own, and work part time.

case *81* *61-Year-Old Male with Gradual Onset of Weakness, Malaise, Orofacial Movements, and Voice Change*

History   A previously healthy 61-year-old male consulted his personal physician for evaluation of a gradual onset of general weakness, malaise, uncontrolled movements of his lower face, and a sensation of clicking in his ears.

Examination   At rest, rhythmic contractions (elevation and depression) of the mandible, faucial arches, soft palate, posterior pharyngeal wall and base of tongue were evident. The musculature was moderately weak, but without atrophy or fasciculations. While assessing the carotid pulse, rhythmic contractions of the extralaryngeal musculature were observed, and occurred in synchrony with movements of the face and velopharynx. Indirect laryngoscopy revealed synchronous contractions of the true and false vocal folds. On forward gaze there was rhythmic vertical occular nystagmus.

Articulation in connected speech was essentially within normal limits, although oral diadochokinetic and sequential motion rates were moderately irregular. Voice quality was moderately harsh with rhythmic changes in volume occurring between 2 and 4 Hz as determined by oscillography. These phonatory features, noted during vowel prolongation, occurred in synchrony with the mandibular, palatal-pharyngeal, and laryngeal contractions.

Respiratory support for speech was considered mildly weak, whereas speaking rate and resonance were essentially within normal limits. Language and oral-speech praxis were within normal limits. Auditory acuity was normal. The clicking noises heard by the patient were also heard by the examiner during the intraoral examination.

Salient symptoms/signs	Test results	Impressions

This worksheet is to be used for recording relevant diagnostic observations. The blank illustration is to be used for identifying and sketching the suspected site of lesion(s). These steps should be completed prior to turning to the Impressions and illustrated site of lesion.

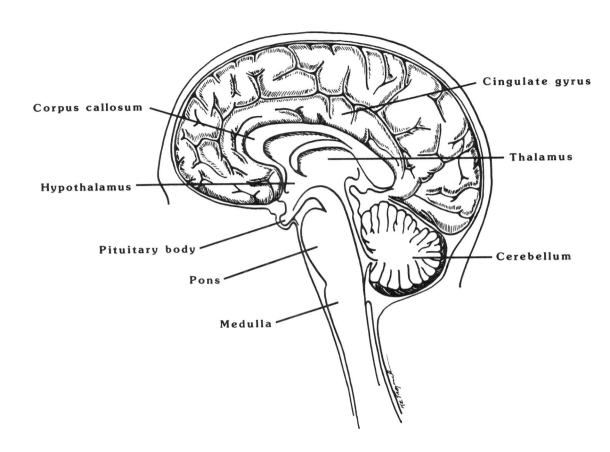

Corpus callosum

Cingulate gyrus

Hypothalamus

Thalamus

Pituitary body

Cerebellum

Pons

Medulla

489   *61-Year-Old Male with Gradual Onset of Weakness, Malaise, Orofacial Movements, and Voice Change*

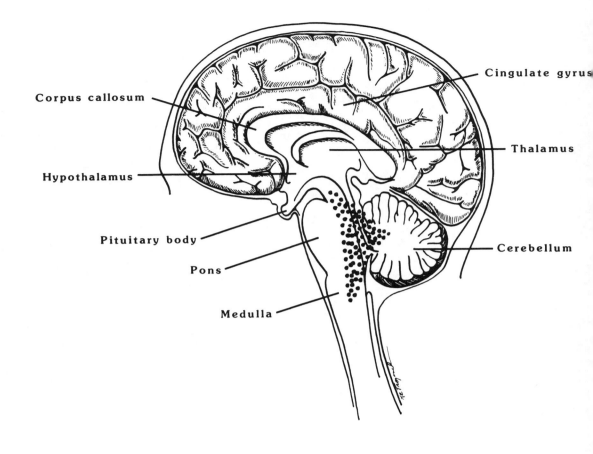

Corpus callosum

Cingulate gyrus

Hypothalamus

Thalamus

Pituitary body

Pons

Cerebellum

Medulla

Impressions   Hyperkinetic (quick) dysarthria; palatal-pharyngeal-laryngeal myoclonus.

Discussion   Lesions involving select areas of the brainstem—in this case a tumor—frequently cause myoclonic movements of the involved musculature. The site of the lesion is thought to be the dentato-rubro-olivary tract (Guillain-Mollaret triangle). The term "myoclonus" in this situation is probably inappropriate in that the movements tend to be regular and rhythmic, occurring typically between 2 and 4 Hz. The term *myoclonus* generally implies abrupt and irregular patterns of movement. Palatal-pharyngeal-laryngeal myoclonus, therefore, may actually be a slow tremor in which rhythmic movements are inherent. The movements are of the resting variety and therefore perceptible primarily during vowel prolongations.

The clicking noises heard by the patient and the examiner were perceptual manifestations of the myoclonic contractions of the involved pharyngeal musculature that control opening and closing of the eustachian tube. Along with tumor, cerebellar infarction, brainstem trauma, and degenerative or demyelinating disease can produce palatal-pharyngeal-laryngeal myoclonus.

History The patient is a 22-year-old male who sustained a closed head injury in a motorcycle accident. He was admitted to hospital in deep coma, which lasted three months. Because of respiratory failure, an emergency tracheotomy had been performed on arrival at the ER. CT scans of the head revealed widespread subdural contusions involving the right cerebral hemisphere and midline brainstem. Because of increasing intracerebral pressure and accumulation of cerebrospinal fluid, he underwent a ventriculo-peritoneal shunt three weeks after admission. The patient's coma eventually resolved. However, he was left with a severe spastic quadriplegia and needed a wheelchair.

Examination Neuropsychological testing at six months after his closed head injury revealed (1) normal to above normal nonverbal intelligence, (2) moderate attention deficits, (3) severe impairment of short-term memory and object recognition, (4) moderately depressed concept formation and cognitive awareness skills, and (5) visuomotor and spatial orientation limitations. Neurolinguistic analyses showed (1) perseverative language strategies, (2) moderate reading comprehension deficits, and (3) mildly impaired auditory verbal comprehension and vocabulary. The oral motor examination revealed (1) bilateral paresis, hypertonicity, discoordination and hyperactive reflexes of the velopharyngeal, lingual, labial, and mandibular musculature; (2) severely imprecise and slow-labored articulation; (3) severe hypernasality and excessive nasal air emissions (greater than 1,000 cc/sec nasal airflow velocities during non-nasal sound productions (normal = 0-100); (4) markedly reduced intra-oral pressure (less than 2 cmH20/5 sec for plosive consonant efforts (normal = 6-8); (5) maximum phonation time at 5 sec (normal = 20); (6) profoundly shortened phrase groups and dysrhythmic/oppositional breathing patterns; (7) Mean glottal airflow rate during phonation at 10 cc/sec (normal = 50-100); (8) glottal resistance at 90 cmH20/lit./sec (normal = 35-50); and (9) severely strained-strangled vocal quality, with associated marked limitations in pitch and loudness control.

493

Salient symptoms/signs	Test results	Impressions

This worksheet is to be used for recording relevant diagnostic observations. The blank illustration is to be used for identifying and sketching the suspected site of lesion(s). These steps should be completed prior to turning to the Impressions and illustrated site of lesion.

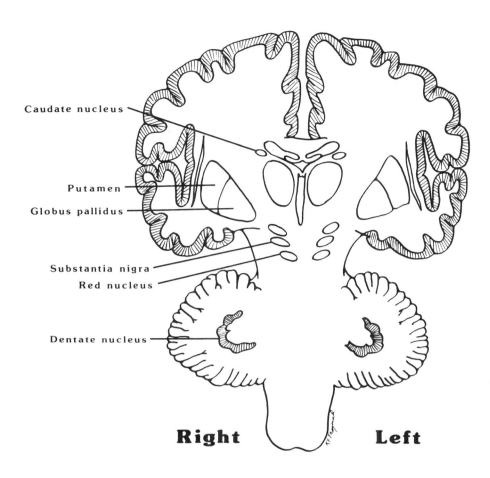

Caudate nucleus

Putamen

Globus pallidus

Substantia nigra

Red nucleus

Dentate nucleus

Right   **Left**

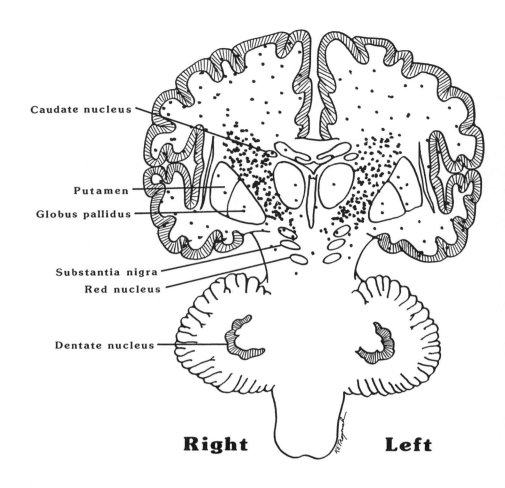

Caudate nucleus

Putamen

Globus pallidus

Substantia nigra
Red nucleus

Dentate nucleus

Right   **Left**

Impressions Spastic dysarthria, severe in degree, concomitant neurocognitive deficits following traumatic brain injury.

Discussion Neurocognitive rehabilitation for this patient stressed short-term memory and spatial orientation, along with visual motor and basic attending skills. Physical and occupational therapy helped the patient with ambulation and to use a walker, perform essential self-help tasks, and learn independent living skills. He underwent a number of surgical procedures to reduce hypertonicity and immobility of the limbs. He had a spinal cord stimulator placed to facilitate limb-trunk musculature activity and coordination. Moderate gains were met in all areas behaviorally and/or surgically treated.

Motor speech intervention first focused on improving respiratory drive and support for speech utilizing exercises for increasing vital capacity, forced expiratory flow rate, and coordinated inhalatory-exhalatory dynamics. For velopharyngeal dysfunction, the patient was fitted with a palatal lift appliance. The respiratory exercises and palatal prosthesis proved moderately successful for increasing respiratory support for speech and reducing hypernasality and nasal emission, respectively.

For the phonatory component of his dysarthria, direct behavioral therapy yielded equivocal results. He was fitted with a portable voice amplification system to facilitate an increase in volume. The appliance allowed for electronic magnification of his voice and, thus, a decrease in effort to be heard.

Articulation therapy incorporated exercises to reduce underlying hypertonicity, weakness, and discoordination of the tongue, lips, and jaw musculature. Phonetic placement exercises were incorporated as the patient demonstrated potential for control. For the slow rate of speech, a metronome and various contrastive stress drills were incorporated to facilitate improvement in the flexibility of his utterances. The formal treatment program lasted approximately 18 months; the patient made progress in all areas treated.

66-Year-Old Male with Progressive Behavioral, Memory, and Language Disturbances

History　Over the course of two years this 66-year-old retired businessman noted progressive difficulty remembering both past and recent events, recalling or using names appropriately, following the gist of conversation, and balancing his checkbook. His spouse denied that he was depressed. He was periodically obstreperous toward family and friends.

Examination　The patient was very cooperative during examination. His speech tended to be verbose, circuitous, and fluent; the content was vague, and semantically incomplete. His vocabulary was reduced and word-finding and naming errors on confrontation were evident. He was frequently echoic to both his own and the examiner's speech. His grammatical skills remained relatively preserved, although occasional sound and word transpositions adversely affected sentence structure. Tests of short- and long-term memory, attention span, visuospatial abilities, and abstract reasoning revealed moderate to severe impairment. Oral speech praxis and neuromuscular functions were felt to be within normal limits.

With the exceptions of mildly elevated blood pressure and hyperactive limb reflexes, the clinical neurological examination proved unremarkable. CT scan suggested enlarged lateral ventricles and generalized cortical atrophy.

Worksheet

Salient symptoms/signs	Test results	Impressions

This worksheet is to be used for recording relevant diagnostic observations. The blank illustration is to be used for identifying and sketching the suspected site of lesion(s). These steps should be completed prior to turning to the Impressions and illustrated site of lesion.

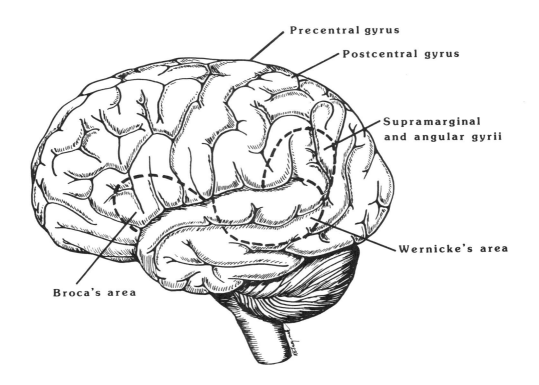

Precentral gyrus

Postcentral gyrus

Supramarginal
and angular gyrii

Wernicke's area

Broca's area

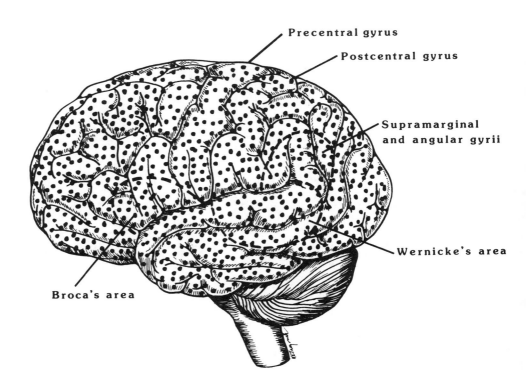

Precentral gyrus

Postcentral gyrus

Supramarginal
and angular gyrii

Wernicke's area

Broca's area

Impressions   Generalized intellectual impairment, dementia of the Alzheimer's type.

Discussion   Alzheimer's disease (AD) is an idiopathic, progressive, currently untreatable, and fatal neurologic disorder suffered by more than 2 million elderly Americans. Confirmatory diagnosis is at autopsy. Proposed causes include: abnormal protein accumulation, reduction in neurotransmitters, and viral agents affecting the central nervous system. Complications associated with the disease result in death, usually within five to ten years. As AD is a gray matter disease, one of its chief debilitating effects is dementia.

Dementia is clinically defined as an acquired disorder characterized by persistent and progressive deterioration of higher intellectual functions, including language, memory, visuospatial skills, and abstract thought. Personality changes are common.

Dementia of the Alzheimer's type must be differentiated from those that are reversible or treatable. Conditions that can produce such dementia include multiple cerebral infarcts, tumors, hydrocephalus, seizures, or vitamin B-12 deficiency. In addition, psychotropic drugs; chronic exposure to lead, mercury, and arsenic and carbon monoxide; as well as protracted use of alcohol, may cause dementia.

The deterioration of cognition, including language, is perhaps the most debilitating sequela to dementia of the Alzheimer type. The initial language signs may be similar to those recognized in focal aphasia, but progress rapidly to involve general cognitive function, including long- and short-term memory particularly.

As the disease progresses, language may become so fragmented that it no longer serves as a useful tool for: (1) communicating with others; (2) conveying or obtaining information; (3) directing actions; (4) making inferences from one's observations; or (5) functioning in daily living.

As with all patients suspected of having AD, the prognosis for our patient was extremely guarded. Speech therapy focused on self-help concepts, naming, and short-term memory.

42-Year-Old Female with Recurrent Stroke

History   This 42-year-old female had suffered her second left cerebral vascular accident eight months previously; the first stroke, which had resulted in minimal deficits occurred more than fifteen years before. The patient had a history of rheumatic and athrosclerotic heart disease; therefore, in each case, a cardio-embolic etiology was presumed. Since her strokes, she complained of a severe left supraorbital headache that tended to linger for as long as one hour. Her medications included enalaprilat (Vasotec), 5 mg. daily; warfarin (Coumadin), 7.5 mg q.i.d., and an iron supplement pill. She had been living alone with family assistance. She was not employed.

On referral from her internist, she presented for comprehensive motor speech, language, and neurologic evaluations. The patient was oriented to time, place, and person and was cooperative throughout all phases of examination.

Examination   On clinical neurologic examination, she exhibited (1) mild weakness of the lower two thirds of the right side of the face, (2) deviation and weakness of the tongue to the right on protrusion without associated atrophy or fasciculations, (3) moderately brisk reflexes of all four limbs with upward going plantar responses bilaterally, (4) mildly depressed general sensation, and (5) mildly discoordinated and slowed gait and balance more pronounced on the right. A CT scan of the head revealed zones of low density in the middle cerebral artery distributions bilaterally, and a focus of low density in the central pons suggestive of a small brainstem infarct. MRI of the head illustrated old bilateral fronto-parietal lobe infarcts and multiple ischemic subcortical white matter lesions within both cerebral hemispheres, greater on the left. The brainstem lesion identified by CT scan was evident as well.

Repeat echocardiography showed left ventricular hypertrophy and mitral valve regurgitation.

Speech and language testing showed moderately halting, imprecise, slow-labored, and repetitive articulatory and prosodic patterns. Inconsistent substitution, omission, and distortion errors were noted, most notably on initial consonants and blends. Cues to slow speaking rate and repeat various utterances yielded improved responses. Nonspeech oral tasks were characterized by groping maneuvers involving the tongue, lips, and jaw; this occurred in the absence of significant neuromuscular impairment. Expressive language was characterized by mild dysnomia, semantic and structural errors contextually. Self-cuing strategies including gestures were used to facilitate verbal output and proved moderately successful for improving the intent of the patient's message. Reading comprehension was mildly impaired. Oral spelling was limited to five-letter words, and short-term memory was moderately deficient. Arithmetic skills showed comparable impairment for both verbal and paper-pencil tasks. Auditory comprehension was mildly impaired.

Salient symptoms/signs	Test results	Impressions

This worksheet is to be used for recording relevant diagnostic observations. The blank illustration is to be used for identifying and sketching the suspected site of lesion(s). These steps should be completed prior to turning to the Impressions and illustrated site of lesion.

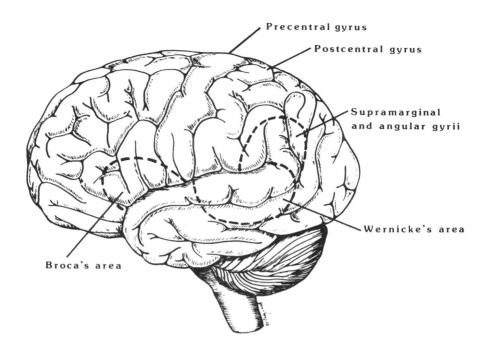

Precentral gyrus

Postcentral gyrus

Supramarginal
and angular gyrii

Wernicke's area

Broca's area

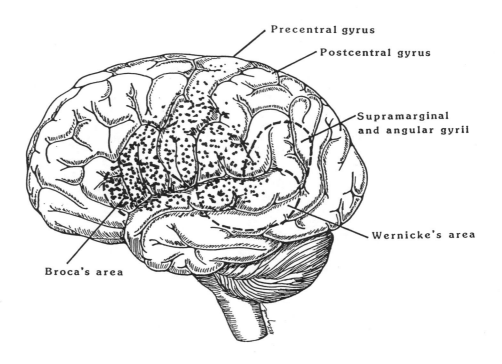

Precentral gyrus

Postcentral gyrus

Supramarginal
and angular gyrii

Wernicke's area

Broca's area

Impressions   Dysphasia, speech-oral dyspraxia complex secondary to recurrent cardiogenic cerebral vascular accidents.

Discussion   This patient exhibited a relatively classic mixture of dysphasia and dyspraxia of speech. The findings from CT and MRI scans offer possible explanations for these motor speech and language disorders. Bifrontal and parietal lobe lesions were evident. The role of the left frontal-parietal areas for motor speech programming and language processing has been well-documented by numerous researchers, as have the adverse affects on communication of pathology in these areas. The signs of limb and orofacial involvement implicate the pyramidal tracts bilaterally.

Our patient had not experienced significant speech or language difficulty following her first CVA 15 years earlier. She had been left, however, with mild right upper extremity weakness. That stroke could be considered mild. Her most recent stroke, however, compounded the residual neurologic deficits (inasmuch as it involved roughly the same areas of the brain as her previous stroke and now created speech and language involvement).

Speech-language therapy stressed the motor speech and language disorders, with occupational and physical therapy directing efforts toward improving tone, strength, force physiology, and coordination of the involved limb and trunk musculature.

At the time of this report, the patient's progress had been slow in all areas, although she remained relatively self-sufficient. Her prognosis for further improvement has been believed to be fair to good, primarily because of her age and determination to succeed.

Bibliography

The following select bibliography represents the authors' attempts to identify and refer the reader to works in the area. Many references are common to more than one diagnostic category.

Aphasia   Alexander, M. et al. Broca's area aphasias. *Neurology.* 40 : 353, 1990.

Bell, W. et al. Neologistic speech automatisms during complex partial seizures. *Neurol.* 40 : 49, 1990.

Benson, D. F. *Aphasia, Alexia, and Agraphia.* New York: Churchill Livingstone, 1979.

Benson, D. F. Aphasia management: The neurologist's role. *Seminars in Speech, Language, and Hearing* 2 : 237, 1981.

Boller, F., Youngjai, K., and Mark, J. L. Auditory Comprehension in Aphasia. In H. Whitaker and H. A. Whitaker, (eds.), *Studies in Neurolinguistics,* Vol. 3. New York: Academic, 1977.

Boller, F. Comprehension disorders in aphasia: A historical review. *Brain Lang.* 5 : 149, 1978.

Brookshire, R. H. (ed.). *Clinical Aphasiology Conference Proceedings.* Minneapolis: BRK Publishers, 1975-1986.

Brookshire, R. H. Auditory Comprehension in Aphasia. In D. F. Johns (ed.), *Clinical Management of Neurogenic Communicative Disorders.* Boston: Little, Brown, 1978.

Brown, J. R. A model for central and peripheral behavior in aphasia. Address to the Annual Meeting of the Academy of Aphasia, Rochester, MN, 1968.

Brown, J. W., and Perecman, E. Neurologic Basis of Language Processing. In J. K. Darby (ed.), *Speech and Language Evaluation in Neurology: Adult Disorders.* New York: Grune & Stratton, 1985.

Cascino, G. et al. Seizure associated in elderly patients. *Mayo Clin Proc.* 66 : 254, 1991.

Caselli, R. J. et al., Rapidly progressive aphasic dementia and motor neuron disease. *Ann Neurol.* 33 : 200, 1993.

Coppens, P. et al. Crossed aphasia: New perspectives. *Aphasiology.* 6 : 585, 1992.

Daffner, K. et al. Broca's aphasia following damage to Wernickes area. *Arch Neurol.* 48 : 766, 1991.

Damasio, A.R. Aphasia. *New Eng J. Med.* 326 : 531, 1992.

Darby, J. K. (ed.). *Speech Evaluation in Medicine.* New York: Grune & Stratton, 1981.

Darley, F. L. *Aphasia.* Philadelphia: Saunders, 1982.

Darley, F. L. Differential Diagnosis of Language Disorders. In F. L. Darley and D. C. Spriestersbach (eds.). *Diagnostic Methods in Speech Pathology* (2nd ed.) New York: Harper & Row, 1978.

Darley, F. L. The efficacy of language rehabilitation in aphasia. *J. Speech Hear. Disord.* 37 : 3, 1972.

Darley, F. L. Treatment of Acquired Aphasia. In W. J. Friedlander (ed.), *Advances in Neurology,* Vol. 7. New York: Raven, 1975.

Darley, F. L. Treat or neglect? *ASHA* 21 : 628, 1979.

DeRenzi, E. and Vignolo, L. A. The Token Test: A sensitive test to detect receptive disturbances in aphasia. *Brain* 85 : 665, 1962.

Duffy, J. R. and Petersen, R. C. Primary progressive aphasia. *Aphasiology.* 6 : 1, 1992.

Gordon, W. P. Neuropsychological Assessment in Aphasia. In J. K. Darby (ed.), *Speech and Language Evaluation in Neurology: Adult Disorders.* New York: Grune & Stratton, 1985.

Halpern, H. *Adult Aphasia.* Indianapolis: Bobbs-Merrill, 1972.

Halpern, H., Darley, F. L., and Brown, J. R. Differential language and neurologic characteristics in cerebral involvement. *J. Speech Hear. Disord.* 38 : 162, 1973.

Harasymiu, S. T., and Halper, A. Sex, age and aphasia type. *Brain Lang.* 12 : 190, 1981.

Hartman, D. E. and Dworkin, J. P. Aphasia, apraxia of speech, and dysarthria. *Gundersen Medical Journal.* 1 : 43, 1993.

Holland, A. (ed.). *Language Disorders in Adults.* San Diego: College-Hill, 1984.

Hooper, L. R., et al. *The Older Aphasic Person.* Rockville, Aspen, 1984.

Jenkins, J. J., Jiminez-Pabon, E., Shaw, R. E., and Sefer, J. W. *Schuell's Aphasia in Adults* (2nd ed.). Hagerstown, Harper & Row, 1975.

Kertesz, A. *Aphasia and Associated Disorders: Taxonomy, Localization and Recovery.* New York: Grune & Stratton, 1979.

Kertesz, A., Harlock, W., and Coates, R. Computer tomographic localization, lesion size, and prognosis in aphasia and nonverbal impairment. *Brain Lang.* 8 : 34, 1979.

Kertesz, A. Recovery of higher cortical functions and therapy. Presented at the American Academy of Neurology, Toronto, Canada, Apr. 1981.

Kertesz, A., and Black, S. E. Cerebrovascular Disease and Aphasia. In J. K. Darby (ed.), *Speech and Language Evaluation in Neurology: Adult Disorders.* New York: Grune & Stratton, 1985.

Kertesz, A., and Sheppard, A. The epidemiology of aphasic and cognitive impairment in stroke. *Brain* 104 : 117, 1981.

LaPointe, L. L. Aphasia Therapy: Some Principles and Strategies for Treatment. In D. F. Johns (ed.), *Clinical Management of Neurogenic Communicative Disorders* (2nd ed.). Boston: Little, Brown, 1985.

LaPoint, L. L. (ed.). Aphasia: Nature and Assessment. *Seminars in Speech and Language,* Vol. 7, 1986.

Lomas, J., and Kertesz, A. Patterns of spontaneous recovery in aphasic groups: A study of adult stroke patients. *Brain Lang.* 5 : 388, 1978.

Mantovani, J. F., and Landau, W. M. Acquired aphasia with convulsive disorder: Course and prognosis. *Neurology* (NY) 30 : 524, 1980.

Marshall, R. et al. Home treatment for aphasic patients by trained nonprofessionals. *J. Speech Hear Dis.* 54 : 462, 1989.

Mayo Clinic and Mayo Foundation. Language and Motor Speech. In *Clinical Examinations in Neurology* (5th ed.). Philadelphia: Saunders, 1981.

McClenahan, R. et al. Misperceptions of comprehension difficulties of stroke patients by doctors, nurses, and relatives. *J. Neurol Neurosurg Psychiat.* 53 : 700, 1990.

Mohr, J. P., et al. Broca aphasia: Pathological and clinical. *Neurology* (NY) 28 : 311, 1978.

Naeser, M. et al. Severe nonfluency in aphasia. *Brain.* 112 : 1, 1989.

Nicholas, M. et al. Aphasia. *Seminars in Speech and Lang.* 11 : 135, 1990.

Obler, L., et al. Aphasia type and aging. *Brain Lang.* 6 : 318, 1978.

O'Connell, P. (ed.). Adult Language Disorders. In K. Butler (ed.), *Topics in Language Disorders,* Vol. 1. Rockville, Aspen, 1981.

Perkins, W. H. (ed.). *Language Handicaps in Adults.* New York: Thieme-Stratton, 1983.

Poeck, K. What do we mean by "aphasic syndrome"? A neurologist's view. *Brain Lang.* 20 : 79, 1983.

Poeck, K. et al. Outcome of intensive language treatment in aphasia. *J. Speech Hear Dis.* 54 : 471, 1989.

Robin, D. et al. Subcortical lesions and aphasia. *J. Speech Hear Dis.* 55 : 90, 1990.

Schuell, H., and Jenkins, J. J. The nature of language deficit in aphasia. *Psychol. Rev.* 66 : 45, 1959.

Serafetinides, E. A., and Falconer, M. A. Speech disturbance in temporal lobe seizures. *Brain* 86 : 333, 1963.

Square-Storer, P. et al. Nonspeech and speech processing skills in patients with aphasia and apraxia of speech. *Brain and Lang.* 33 : 33, 1988.

Tompkins, C. et al. On prognostic research in adult neurologic disorders. *J. Speech Hear Res.* 33 : 398, 1990.

Wertz, R. T. Neuropathologies of Speech and Language: An Introduction to Patient Management. In D. F. Johns (ed.), *Clinical Management of Neurogenic Communicative Disorders* (2nd ed.). Boston: Little, Brown, 1985.

Apraxia of Speech

Abbs, J. H., and Rosenbek, J. C. Some Motor Control Perspectives on Apraxia of Speech and Dysarthria. In J. Costello (ed.), *Recent Advances in Speech Disorders in Adults.* San Diego: College-Hill, 1984.

Aten, J. L., et al. *Letter:* Comment on A.D. Martin's "Some objections to the term apraxia of speech." *J. Speech Hear. Dis.* 40 : 416, 1975.

Brookshire, R. H. (ed.). *Clinical Aphasiology Conference Proceedings.* Minneapolis: BRK Publishers, 1975-1986.

Buckingham, H. W. Explanations in apraxia with consequences for the concept of apraxia of speech. *Brain Lang.* 8 : 202, 1979.

Canter, G., et al. Contrasting speech patterns in apraxia of speech and phonemic paraphasia. *Brain Lang.* 20 : 204, 1985.

Clarke, C.E. et al. Cerebral localization in articulatory dyspraxia. *J. Neurol Neurosurg Psychiat.* 55 : 168, 1992.

Critchley, M. Articulatory defects in aphasia. *J. Laryngol. Otol.* 66 : 1, 1952.

Darley, F. L. *Aphasia.* Philadelphia: Saunders, 1982.

Darley, F. L. Differential Diagnosis of Acquired Motor Speech Disorders. In F. L. Darley and D. C. Spriestersbach (eds.), *Diagnostic Methods in Speech Pathology* (2nd ed.). New York: Harper & Row, 1978.

Darley, F. L., Aronson, A. E., and Brown, J. R. *Motor Speech Disorders.* Philadelphia: Saunders, 1975.

Darley, F. L., Aronson, A. E., and Brown, J. R. *Motor Speech Disorders: Audio Seminars in Speech Pathology.* Philadelphia: Saunders, 1975.

Deal, J. L., and Darley, F. L. The influences of linguistic and situational variables in phonemic accuracy in apraxia of speech. *J. Speech Hear. Res.* 15 : 639, 1972.

DeRenzi, E., et al. Oral apraxia and aphasia. *Cortex* 2 : 50, 1972.

Dworkin, J. P., Abkarian, G. G., and Johns, D. F. Apraxia of speech: the effectiveness of a treatment regimen. *J. Speech Hear. Disord.* 53 : 280, 1988.

Geschwind, N. The apraxias: Neural mechanisms of disorders of learned movement. *Am. Sci.* 63 : 188, 1975.

Guyette, T. W., and Diedrich, W. M. A Critical Review of Developmental Apraxia of Speech. In N. Lass (ed.), *Speech and Language: Advances in Basic Research and Practice,* New York: Academic Press 1981.

Halpern, H., Darely, F. L., and Brown, J. R. Differential language and neurologic characteristics in cerebral involvement. *J. Speech Hear. Disord.* 78 : 162, 1973.

Heilman, K. M. Apraxia. In K. M. Heilman and E. Valenstein (eds.), *Clinical Neuropsychology.* New York: Oxford University Press, 1979.

Itoh, M., et al. Abnormal articulatory dynamics in a patient with apraxia of speech: X-ray microbeam observation. *Brain Lang.* 11 : 66, 1980.

Itoh, M., et al. Velar movements during speech in a patient with apraxia of speech. *Brain Lang.* 7 : 227, 1979.

Itoh, M., et al. Voice onset time characteristics in apraxia of speech. *Brain Lang.* 17 : 193, 1982.

Johns, D. F., and Darley, F. L. Phonemic variability in apraxia of speech. *J. Speech Hear. Res.* 13 : 556, 1970.

Johns, D. F., and LaPointe, L. L. Neurogenic Disorders of Output Processing: Apraxia of Speech. In H. Whitaker and H. A. Whitaker (eds.), *Studies in Neurolinguistics,* Vol. 1. New York: Academic, 1976.

Kelso, J. A., and Tuller, B. Toward a theory of apractic syndromes. *Brain Lang.* 12 : 224, 1981.

Kirshner, H. Apraxia of speech: A linguistic enigma: (A neurologist's perspective). In W. Webb (ed.), *Seminars in Speech and Language.* 13, 14, 1992.

LaPointe, L. L., and Johns, D. F. Some phonemic characteristics of apraxia in speech. *J. Commun. Disord.* 8 : 259, 1975.

LaPointe, L. L., and Wertz, R. T. Oral movement abilities and articulatory characteristics of brain-injured adults. *Percept. Mot. Skills.* 39 : 39, 1974.

Marshall, R. et al. Selective impairment of phonation: A case study. *Brain and Lang.* 35 : 313, 1988.

Martin, A. D. Some objections to the term apraxia of speech. *J. Speech Hear. Disord.* 39 : 53, 1974.

Martin, A. D. Letter: Reply to Aten, Darley, Deal and Johns. *J. Speech Hear. Disord.* 40 : 420, Erratum, p. 549 (1975).

Mateer, L., et al. Impairment of nonverbal oral movements in apraxia. *Brain Lang.* 4 : 202, 1977.

Mayo Clinic and Mayo Foundation. Language and Motor Speech. In *Clinical Examinations in Neurology* (5th ed.). Philadelphia: Saunders, 1981.

Miller, N. *Dyspraxia and its Management.* Rockville, Aspen, 1986.

Mlcoch, A. G., and Noll, J. D. Speech production models as related to the concept of apraxia of speech. In N. J. Lass (ed.), *Speech and Language: Advances in Basic Research and Practice.* New York: Academic, 1980.

Mohr, J. P., et al. Broca aphasia: Pathologic and clinical. *Neurology* 28 : 311, 1978.

Perkins, W. (ed.). *Dysarthria and Apraxia.* New York: Thieme-Stratton, 1983.

Rosenbek, J. C., McNeil, M. R., and Aronson, A. L. *Apraxia of Speech: Physiology, Acoustics, Linguistics, Management.* San Diego: College-Hill, 1984.

Rosenbek, J. C., Wertz, R. T., and Darley, F. L. Oral sensation and perception in apraxia of speech and aphasia. *J. Speech Hear. Res.* 16 : 22, 1973.

Rosenbek, J. C. Treating Apraxia of Speech. In D. F. Johns (ed.), *Clinical Management of Neurogenic Communicative Disorders* (2nd ed.). Boston: Little, Brown, 1985.

Sarno, M. T. *Acquired Aphasia.* New York: Academic, 1981.

Shankweiler, D., and Harris, K. S. An experimental approach to the problem of articulation in aphasia. *Cortex* 49 : 277, 1966.

Shewan, C. M. Verbal dyspraxia and its treatment. *Human Commun.* 5 : 3, 1980.

Square-Storer, P. et al. An acoustic study of apraxia of speech in patients with different lesion loci. In C. Moore, K. Yorkston, and D. Beukelman (eds.), *Recent Advances in Motor Speech Disorders.* San Diego, College-Hill Press, 1991.

Tognola, G., and Vignolo, L. Brain lesions associated with oral apraxia in stroke patients: a clinico-neuroradiological investigation with the CT scan. *Neuropsychologica* 18 : 257, 1980.

Trost, J. E., and Canter, G. J. Apraxia of speech in patients with Broca's aphasia: A study of phonemic production accuracy and error patterns. *Brain Lang.* 1 : 63, 1974.

Wertz, R. T., et al. A review of 228 cases of apraxia of speech: Classification, etiology, and localization. Presented at the Annual Meeting of the American Speech and Hearing Association, New York, New York, 1970.

Wertz, R. T., LaPointe, L. L., and Rosenbek, J. C. *Apraxia of Speech in Adults: The Disorder and Its Management.* New York: Grune & Stratton, 1984.

Wertz, R. T. Neuropathologies of Speech and Language: An Introduction to Patient Management. In D. F. Johns (ed.), *Clinical Management of Neurogenic Communicative Disorders* (2nd ed.). Boston: Little, Brown, 1985.

Confused Language

Adamovitch, B. B., and Henderson, J. Treatment of Communication Deficits Resulting from Traumatic Head Injury. In W. H. Perkins (ed.), *Current Therapy of Communication Disorders.* New York: Thieme-Stratton, 1983.

Adamovich, B. and Henderson, J. *Scales of Cognitive Ability for Traumatic Brain Injury.* Boston: Riverside Publishing, 1992.

Berrol, S. Issues in cognitive rehabilitation. *Arch Neurol.* 47 : 219, 1990.

Chedru, F., and Geschwind, N. Disorders of higher cortical functions in acute confusional states. *Cortex* 8 : 395, 1972.

Darby, J. K. (ed.). *Speech Evaluation in Medicine.* New York: Grune & Stratton, 1981.

Darley, F. L. *Aphasia.* Philadelphia: Saunders, 1982.

Groher, M. Language and memory disorders following closed head trauma. *J. Speech Hear. Res.* 20 : 212, 1977.

Halpern, H., et al. Differential language and neurologic characteristics in cerebral involvement. *J. Speech Hear. Disord.* 38 : 162, 1973.

Heilman, K. M., et al. Closed head trauma and aphasia. *J. Neurol. Neurosurg. Psychiatry* 34 : 265, 1971.

Holland, A. (ed.). *Language Disorders in Adults.* San Diego: College-Hill, 1984.

Hooper, R. *Patterns of Acute Head Injury.* Baltimore: Williams & Wilkins, 1969.

Howard, M., et al. *A Manual of Behavior Management Strategies for Traumatically Brain Injured Adults.* Chicago: Rehabilitation Institute of Chicago, 1983.

Jennett, B., and Teasdale, G. *Management of Head Injuries.* Philadelphia: Davis, 1981.

Langfitt, T. W. Measuring the outcome from head injuries. *J. Neurosurg.* 48 : 673, 1978.

Levin, H. S., et al. *Neurobehavioral Consequences of Closed Head Injury.* New York: Oxford University Press, 1982.

Levin, H. S., et al. Aphasic disorders in patients with closed head injury. *J. Neurol. Neurosurg. Psychiatry* 39 : 1062, 1976.

Levin, H. S., and Grossman, R. G. Behavioral sequelae of closed head injury: A quantitative study. *Arch. Neurol.* 35 : 720, 1978.

Levin, H. S., et al. Linguistic recovery after closed head injury. *Brain Lang.* 12 : 360, 1981.

Levin, H. S., et al. Long-term neuropsychological outcome of closed head injury. *J. Neurosurg.* 50 : 412, 1979.

Levin, H. S., and Esenberg, H. M. Neuropsychological impairment after closed head injury in children and adolescents. *J. Pediatr. Psychol.* 4 : 389, 1979.

Levin, W. Rehabilitation after head injury. *Br. Med. J.* 1 : 465, 1968.

Levin, W. *The Management of Head Injuries.* Baltimore: Williams & Wilkins, 1966.

Lezak, M. D. Recovery of memory and learning functions following traumatic brain injury. *Cortex* 15 : 63, 1979.

Lishman, W. A. The psychiatric sequelae of head injury: A review. *Psychol. Med.* 3 : 304, 1973.

Luria, A. R. *Traumatic Aphasia: Its Syndromes, Psychology and Treatment.* The Hague: Mouton, 1970.

Mandleberg, I. A., and Brooks, D. N. Cognitive retraining after severe head injury. I. Serial testing on the Wechsler Adult Intelligence Scale. *J. Neurol. Neurosurg. Psychiatry* 38 : 1121, 1975.

Mayo Clinic and Mayo Foundation. Language and Motor Speech. In *Clinical Examinations in Neurology* (5th ed.). Philadelphia: Saunders, 1981.

Mesulam, M. M., et al. Acute confusional states with right middle cerebral artery infarctions. *J. Neurol. Neurosurg. Psychiatry* 39 : 84, 1976.

Miller, E. The training characteristics of severely head-injured patients: A preliminary study. *J. Neurol. Neurosurg. Psychiatry* 43 : 525, 1980.

Miller, J. D., et al. Further experiences in the management of severe head injury. *J. Neurosurg.* 54 : 289, 1981.

Millikan, L. H., and Darley, F. L. (eds.). *Brain Mechanisms Underlying Speech and Language.* New York: Grune & Stratton, 1967.

Popp, A. J., et al. (eds.). *Neural Trauma.* New York: Raven, 1979.

Sarno, M. T. The nature of verbal impairment after closed head injury. *J. Nerv. Ment. Dis.* 1 68 : 685, 1979.

Shapiro, B. E., et al. Mechanisms of confabulation. *Neurology* 31 : 1070, 1981.

Stuss, D. T., et al. An extraordinary form of confabulation. *Neurology* (NY) 28 : 1166, 1978.

Sweet, R. L., et al. Significance of bilateral abnormalities on the CT scan in patients with severe head injury. *Neurosurgery* 3 : 16, 1978.

Thomsen, I. V. Evaluation and outcome of aphasia in patients with severe closed head trauma. *J. Neurol. Neurosurg. Psychiatry* 38 : 713, 1975.

Thomsen, I. V. Evaluation and outcome of traumatic aphasia in patients with severe focal lesions. *Folia Phoniatr. (Basel)* 28 : 362, 1976.

Walker, A. E., and Critchley, M. (eds.). *The Late Effects of Head Injury.* Springfield, IL: Thomas, 1969.

Vapalahti, M., and Troup, H. Prognosis for patients with severe brain injuries. *Br. Med. I.* 3 : 404, 1971.

Weinstein, E. A., et al. Linguistic patterns of misnaming in brain injury. *Neuropsychologica* 1 : 79, 1963.

Weinstein, E. A., et al. Confabulation following brain injury. *Arch. Gen. Psychiatry* 18 : 348, 1968.

Wertz, R. T. Neuropathologies of Speech and Language: An Introduction to Patient Management. In D. F. Johns (ed.), *Clinical Management of Neurogenic Communicative Disorders* (2nd ed.). Boston: Little, Brown, 1985.

Ylvisaker, M., and Holland, A. Coaching, self-coaching and rehabilitation of head injury. In D. F. Johns (ed.), *Clinical Management of Neurogenic Communicative Disorders* (2nd ed.). Boston: Little, Brown, 1985.

Generalized Intellectual Impairment

Appell, J., et al. A study of language functioning in Alzheimer patients. *Brain Lang.* 17 : 73, 1982.

Appel, S. H. A unifying hypothesis for the cause of amyotrophic lateral sclerosis. Parkinsonism, and Alzheimer's disease. *Ann Neurol.* 10 : 495, 1981.

Baratz, R., and Herzog, A. G. The communication disorder in dialysis dementia: A case report. *Brain Lang.* 10 : 378, 1980.

Bayles, K. A. Language function in senile dementia. *Brain Lang.* 16 : 265, 1982.

Bayles, K. A., and Boone, D. R. The potential of language tasks for identifying senile dementia. *J. Speech Hear. Disord.* 47 : 210, 1982.

Berg, L., et al. Predictive features in mild senile dementia of the Alzheimer's type. *Neurology* 34 : 563, 1984.

Boller, F., et al. Parkinson's disease, dementia, and Alzheimer's disease: Clinicopathological correlations. *Ann. Neurol.* 7 : 329, 1980.

Cummings, J. L., et al. Aphasia in dementia of the Alzheimer's type. *Neurology* 35 : 394, 1985.

Cummings, J. L., and Benson, D. F. *Dementia: a clinical approach.* Boston: Butterworth, 1983.

Cummings, J. L., and Benson, D. F. Subcortical dementia: Review of an emerging concept. *Arch. Neurol.* 41 : 874, 1984.

Darby, J. K. (ed.). *Speech Evaluation in Medicine.* New York: Grune & Stratton, 1981.

Darley, F. L. *Aphasia.* Philadelphia: Saunders, 1982.

de Ajuriaguerra, J., and Tissot, R. Some Aspects of Language in Various Forms of Senile De mentia. In E. H. Lenneberg and E. Lenneberg (eds.), *Foundations of Language Development.* New York: Academic, 1975.

Eslinger, P.J. Neuropsychologic detection of abnormal mental decline in older persons. *J.A.M.A.* 253 : 670, 1985.

Foley, J. M. Differential Diagnosis of the Organic Mental Disorders in Elderly Patients. In L. M. Gaitz (ed.), *Aging and the Brain.* New York: Plenum, 1972.

Garron, D. C., et al. Intellectual functioning of persons with idiopathic Parkinsonism. *J. Nerv. Ment. Dis.* 154 : 445, 1972.

Gustafson, L., et al. Speech disturbances in presenile dementia related to local blood flow abnormalities in the brain. *Brain Lang.* 5 : 103, 1978.

Hachinski, V. L., et al. Multi-farct dementia: A cause of mental deterioration in the elderly. *Lancet* 2 : 207, 1974.

Halpern, H., et al. Differential language and neurological characteristics in cerebral involvement. *J. Speech Hear. Disord.* 38 : 162, 1973.

Holland, A. (ed.). *Language Disorders in Adults.* San Diego: College-Hill, 1984.

Hooper, C. R., et al. *The Older Aphasic Person.* Rockville, Aspen, 1984.

Hutton, J. T. (ed.). *Dementia* (Neurologic Clinics, Vol. 4). Philadelphia: Saunders, 1986.

Katzman, R. Early detection of senile dementia. *Hosp. Pract.* June, 61, 1981.

Katzman, R. Dementia. In S. H. Appel (ed.), *Current Neurology,* Vol. 5. New York: Wiley, 1984.

Katzman, R., Terry, R. D., and Bicks, K. L. (eds.). *Alzheimer's Disease: Senile Dementia and Related Disorders.* New York: Raven, 1978.

Kirshner, H. S., et al. Language disturbance: An initial symptom of cortical degeneration and dementia. *Arch. Neurol.* 41 : 491, 1984.

Kerzner, L. J. Diagnosis and Treatment of Alzheimer's Disease. In G. H. Stollerman (ed.), *Advances in Internal Medicine.* Chicago: Year Book, 1984.

Kokmen, E. et al., A short test of mental status: Description and preliminary results. *Mayo Clinic Proceed.* 62 : 281, 1987.

Kontiola, P. et al. Pattern of language impairment is different in Alzheimer's Disease and multi-infarct dementia. *Brain and Lang.* 38 : 364, 1990.

Loewenstein, D.A. et al. Predominant left hemisphere metabolic dysfunction in dementia. *Arch Neurol.* 46 : 146, 1989.

Mackay, L. et al. Early intervention in sever head injury: Long term benefits of a formalized program. *Arch Phys Med Rehab.* 73 : 635, 1992.

Madison, D. P., et al. Communicative and cognitive deterioration in dialysis dementia: Two case studies. *J. Speech Hear. Disord.* 42 : 238, 1977.

Martin, W. E., et al. Parkinson's disease: Clinical analysis of 100 patients. *Neurology* 23 : 783, 1973.

Mayeux, R., et al. Is "subcortical dementia" a recognizable clinical entity? *Ann. Neurol.* 14 : 278, 1983.

Mayeux, R., et al. Heterogeneity in dementia of the Alzheimer type: Evidence of subgroups. *Neurology* 35 : 453, 1985.

Mayo Clinic and Mayo Foundation. Language and Motor Speech. In *Clinical Examinations in Neurology* (5th ed.). Philadelphia: Saunders, 1981.

McKhann, G., et al. Clinical diagnosis of Alzheimer's disease: Report of the NINCDS-ADRDA work group. *Neurology* 34 : 939, 1984.

Miller, N. E., and Cohen, G. D. (eds.). *Clinical Aspects of Alzheimer's Disease and Senile Dementia.* New York: Raven, 1981.

Molsa, P., et al. Validity of clinical diagnosis in dementia: a perspective clinicopathologic study. *J. Neurol. Neurosurg. Psychiatry* 48 : 1085, 1985.

Murray, J., et al. Differential diagnosis of aphasia and dementia from aphasia test battery scores. *J. Neurol. Comm. Dis.* 1 : 33, 1983.

Obler, L. K. Language and brain dysfunction in dementia. In S. Segalowitz (ed.), *Language Functions and Brain Organization.* New York: Academic, 1977.

Obler, L. K., and Albert, M. L. Language in the elderly aphasic and in the dementing patient. In M. T. Sarno (ed.), *Acquired Aphasia.* New York: Academic, 1981.

Perkins, W. H. (ed.). *Language Handicaps in Adults.* New York: Thieme-Stratton, 1983.

Schwartz, M. F., et al. Dissociations of language function in dementia: A case study. *Brain Lang.* 7 : 277, 1979.

Seltzer, B., and Sherwin, I. A comparison of clinical features in early and late onset primary degenerative dementia. *Arch. Neurol.* 40 : 143, 1983.

Smith, W. L., and Kinsbourne, M. (eds.). *Aging and Dementia.* New York: Spectrum, 1977.

Storandt, M., et al. Psychometric differentiation of mild senile dementia of the Alzheimer type. *Arch. Neurol.* 41 : 197, 1985.

Terry, R. D., and Katzman, R. Senile dementia of the Alzheimer type. *Ann. Neurol.* 14 : 497, 1983.

Tomoeda, C.K. et al. The efficacy of speech-language pathology intervention: Dementia. *Seminars in Speech and Language.* 11 : 311, 1990.

Watson, J. M., and Records, L. E. The effectiveness of the Porch Index of Communicative Ability as a diagnostic tool in assessing specific behaviors of senile dementia. In R. Brookshire (ed.), *Clinical Aphasiology.* Minneapolis: BRK Publishers, 1978.

Wertz, R. T. Neuropathologies of Speech and Language: An Introduction to Patient Management. In D. F. Johns (ed.), *Clinical Management of Neurogenic Communicative Disorders* (2nd ed.). Boston: Little, Brown, 1985.

Wisniewski, K. E. Occurrence of neuropathological changes and dementia of Alzheimer's disease in Down's syndrome. *Ann. Neurol.* 17 : 278, 1985.

Dysarthria   Abbs, J. H., and Rosenbek, J. C. Some Motor Control Perspectives on Apraxia of Speech and Dysarthria. In J. Costello (ed.), *Speech Disorders in Adults: Recent Advances.* San Diego: College-Hill, 1985.

Aronson, A. E. Dysarthria. In T. J. Hixon, L. D. Shriberg, and J. H. Saxman (eds.), *Introduction to Communicative Disorders.* Englewood Cliffs, NJ: Prentice-Hall, 1980.

Barlow, S., and Abbs, J. Force transclucers for the evaluation of labial, lingual, and mandibular motor impairments. *J. Speech Hear. Disord.* 26 : 616, 1983.

Bassich, C. J., et al. Speech symptoms associated with early signs of Shy-Drager syndrome. *J. Neurol. Neurosurg. Psychiatry* 47 : 995, 1984.

Berry, W. R. (ed.). *Clinical Dysarthria.* San Diego: College-Hill, 1983.

Berry, W. R., et al. Dysarthria in Wilson's disease. *J. Speech Hear. Res.* 17 : 169, 1974.

Berry, W. R., et al. Effects of penicillamine therapy and low copper diet on dysarthria in Wilson's disease (hepatolenticular degeneration). *Mayo Clin. Proc.* 49 : 405, 1974.

Beukelman, D., and Yorkston, K. A communication system for the severely dysarthric speaker with an intact language system. *J. Speech Hear. Disord.* 42 : 265, 1977.

Beukelman, D. R., and Yorkston, K. M. The relationship between information transfer and speech intelligibility of dysarthric speakers. *J. Commun. Disord.* 12 : 188, 1979.

Boller, F., et al. Palilalia. Br. *J. Disord. Commun.* 10 : 92, 1975.

Brown, J. R., Darley, F. L., and Aronson, A. E. Ataxic dysarthria. *Int. J. Neurol.* 7 : 302, 1970.

Canter, G. J. Neuromotor pathologies of speech. *Am. J. Phys. Med.* 46 : 659, 1967.

Canter, G. J. Observations on neurogenic stuttering: A contribution to differential diagnosis. *Br. J. Disord. Commun.* 6 : 139, 1971.

Canter, G. J. Speech characteristics of patients with Parkinson's disease. I. Intensity, pitch, and duration. *J. Speech Hear. Disord.* 28 : 221, 1963.

Canter, G. J. Speech characteristics of patients with Parkinson's disease. II. Physiological support for speech. *J. Speech Hear. Disord.* 30 : 44, 1965.

Canter, G. J. Speech characteristics of patients with Parkinson's disease. III. Articulation, diadochokinesis and overall speech adequacy. *J. Speech Hear. Disord.* 30 : 217, 1965.

Carrow, E., et al. Deviant speech characteristics of motor neuron disease. *Arch. Otolaryngol.* 100 : 212, 1974.

Critchley, E. M. R. Speech disorders of Parkinsonism: A review. *J. Neurol. Neurosurg. Psychiatry* 44 : 751, 1981.

Darby, J. K. (ed.). *Speech Evaluation in Medicine.* New York: Grune & Stratton, 1981.

Darley, F. L., Aronson, A. E., and Brown, J. R. Differential diagnostic patterns of dysarthria. *J. Speech Hear. Res.* 12 : 224, 1969.

Darley, F. L., Aronson, A. E., and Brown, J. R. Clusters of deviant speech dimensions in the dysarthrias. *J. Speech Hear. Res.* 12 : 462, 1969.

Darley, F. L., Brown, J. R., and Goldstein, N. P. Dysarthria in multiple sclerosis. *J. Speech Hear. Res.* 15 : 229, 1972.

Darley, F. L., Aronson, A. E., and Brown, J. R. *Motor Speech Disorders: Audio Seminars in Speech Pathology.* Philadelphia: Saunders, 1975.

Darley, F. L., Aronson, A. E., and Brown, J. R. *Motor Speech Disorders.* Philadelphia: Saunders, 1975.

Darley, F. L. Differential Diagnosis of Acquired Motor Speech Disorders. In
F. L. Darley and D. C. Spriestersbach (eds.), *Diagnostic Methods in Speech
Pathology* (2nd ed.). New York: Harper & Row, 1978.

Dworkin, J. P. *Motor Speech Disorders: A Treatment Guide.* St. Louis : Mosby,
1991.

Dworkin, J. P., and Johns, D. F. Management of velopharyngeal incompetence
in dysarthria: A historical review. *Clin. Otolaryngol.* 5 : 61, 1980.

Enderby, P. Long term recovery patterns of severe dysarthria following head
injury. *Brit J. Dis Com.* 25 : 341, 1991.

Gentil, M. Dysarthria in Friedreich's Disease. *Brain and Lang.* 38 : 438, 1990.

Gerratt, B. R., et al. Speech abnormalities in tardive dyskinesia. *Arch. Neurol.*
41 : 273, 1984.

Golper, L. H., et al. Focal cranial dystonia. *J. Speech Hear. Disord.* 2 : 128,
1983.

Grewel, F. Classifications of dysarthrias. *Acta. Psychiatr. Neurol. Scand.* 32 :
325, 1957.

Hardy, J. L. Suggestions for physiologic research in dysarthria. *Cortex* 3 : 128,
1967.

Hartman, D. E. Neurogenic dysphonia. *Ann. Otol. Rhinol. Laryngol.* 93 : 57,
1984.

Hartman, D. E., and Abbs, J. A. The Dysarthrias of Movement Disorders. In
J. Jankovic and E. Tolsa (eds.), *Facial Dyskinesias* (Advances in Neurology).
New York: Raven 49 : 289, 1988.

Hartman, D. E. and Abbs, J. H. Dysarthria associated with focal unilateral
upper motor neuron lesion. *European J. Dis Com.* 27 : 187, 1992.

Hartman, D. E. and O'Neill, B. P. Progressive dysfluency, dysphagia, dysarthria:
A case of olivoponto cerebellar atrophy. In Yorkston, K. and Beukelman,
D. (eds.). *Recent Advances in Clinical Dysarthria.* San Diego: College-Hill
Press, 1989.

Hartman, D. E. et al. Response of essential voice tremor and spasmodic
dysphonia of essential voice tremor to methazolamide (Neptazaen). In
press.

Hunker, C., et al. The relationship between Parkinsonism rigidity and
hypokinesia in the orofacial system: A quantitative analysis. *Neurology* 32
: 755, 1982.

Jankovich, J. (ed.). Movement Disorders. *Neurologic Clinics* Vol. 2,
Philadelphia: Saunders, 1984.

Joanette, Y., et al. Dysarthria symptomatology of Friedreich's ataxia. *Brain
Lang.* 10 : 39, 1980.

Johns, D. F. Surgical and Prosthetic Management of Neurogenic Velopharyngeal Incompetency in Dysarthria. In D. F. Johns (ed.), *Clinical Management
of Neurogenic Communicative Disorders* (2nd ed.). Boston, Little, Brown,
1985.

Kent, R. D., and Netsell, R. Articulatory abnormalities in athetoid cerebral
palsy. *J. Speech Hear. Disord.* 43 : 353, 1978.

Kent, R. D., Netsell, R., and Abbs, J. H. Acoustic characteristics of dysarthria
associated with cerebellar disease. *J. Speech Hear. Res.* 22 : 627, 1979.

Kent, R., and Rosenbek, J. Prosodic disturbance and neurologic lesions. *Brain
Lang.* 15 : 259, 1982.

Koller, W. L. Dysfluency (stuttering) in extrapyramidal disease. *Arch. Neurol.*
40 : 175, 1983.

Koller, W. L. Edentulous orodyskinesia. *Ann. Neurol.* 13 : 97, 1983.

La Pointe, L. L. and Horner, J. Palilalia: A descriptive study of pathological
reiterative utterances. *J. Speech Hear Dis.* 46 : 34, 1981.

Lechtenberg, R., and Gilman, S. Speech disorders in cerebellar disease. *Ann. Neurol.* 3 : 285, 1978.

Lefkowitz, D. and Netsell, R. Neuroanatomy of speech: An MRI atlas. *J. Med Speech-Language Path.* 1 : 3, 1993.

Linebaugh, D. The dysarthria of Shy-Drager syndrome. *J. Speech Hear Disord.* 44 : 55, 1979.

Logemann, J., et al. Frequency and co-occurrence of vocal tract dysfunction in speech of a large sample of Parkinson's patients. *J. Speech Hear. Disord.* 43 : 47, 1978.

Logemann, J., and Fischer, H. Vocal tract control in Parkinson's disease Phonetic feature analyses of misarticulations. *J. Speech Hear. Disord.* 46 : 348, 1981.

Ludlow, C. Treatment of speech and voice disorders with botulinum toxin. *JAMA.* 28 : 2671, 1990.

Ludlow, C. L., Bassich, C. J., and Connor, N. P. An Objective System for Assessment and Analysis of Dysarthric Speech. In J. K. Darby (ed.), *Speech and Language Evaluation in Neurology: Adult Disorders.* New York: Grune & Stratton, 1985.

Marsden, C. D. The anatomical basis of symptomatic hemidystonia. *Brain,* 108, 463, 1985.

Mayo Clinic and Mayo Foundation. Language and Motor Speech. In *Clinical Examinations in Neurology* (5th ed.). Philadelphia: Saunders, 1981.

McNeil, M. R., Rosenbek, J. L., and Aronson, A. E. (eds.). *The Dysarthrias: Physiology, Acoustics, Perception, Management.* San Diego: College-Hill, 1984.

McNeil, M. et al. Oral structure nonspeech motor control in normal, dysarthric, aphasic, and apraxic speakers: Isometric force and static position control. *J. Speech Hear Res.* 33 : 255, 1990.

Mueller, P. B. Parkinson's disease: Motor-speech behavior in a selected group of patients. *Folia Phoniatr.* 23 : 333, 1971.

Muenter, M. et al. Treatment of essential tremor with Methazolamide. *Mayo Clin Proc.* 66 : 991, 1991.

Neilson, P., et al. Pathophysiology of dysarthria in cerebral palsy. *J. Neurol. Neurosurg. Psychiatry* 44 : 1013, 1981.

Netsell, R., et al. Acceleration and weakness in Parkinson's dysarthria. *J. Speech Hear. Disord.* 40 : 170, 1975.

Netsell, R., and Daniel, B. Dysarthria in adults: Physiologic approach to rehabilitation. *Arch. Phys. Med. Rehabil.* 60 : 502, 1979.

Netsell, R. Speech Motor Control and Selective Neurologic Disorders. In S. Grillner, et al. (eds.), *Speech Motor Control.* Elmsford, NY: Pergamon, 1982.

Perkins, W. H. (ed.). *Dysarthria and Apraxia.* New York: Thieme-Stratton, 1983.

Platt, L., et al. Dysarthria of adult cerebral palsy. I. Intelligibility and articulatory impairment. *J. Speech Hear. Disord.* 23 : 28, 1980.

Platt, L. J., et al. Dysarthria of adult cerebral palsy. II. Phonemic analysis of articulation errors. *J. Speech Hear. Disord.* 23 : 41, 1980.

Portnoy, R. A. Hyperkinetic dysarthria as an early indicator of impending tardive dyskinesia. *J. Speech Hear. Disord.* 44 : 214, 1979.

Rosenbek, J. C. (ed.). Current Views of Dysarthria. In W. Perkins (ed.), *Seminars in Speech and Language,* Vol. 5. New York: Thieme-Stratton, 1984.

Rosenfield, D. B., and Kinsbourne, M. Neurobehavior. In S. H. Appel (ed.), *Current Neurology,* Vol. 5. New York: Wiley, 1984.

Sapir, S. and Aronson, A. E. Co-existing psychogenic and neurogenic dysphonia: A source of diagnostic confusion. *Brit J. Dis Commun.,* 22 : 73, 1987.

Sarno, M. Speech impairment in Parkinson's disease. *Arch. Phys. Med. Rehabil.* 49 : 269, 1968.

Sataloff, R. T. (ed.) Spasmodic dysphonia. *J. Voice.* 6 : 293, 1992.

Shawker, T. H., and Sonies, B. C. Tongue movements during speech: A real time ultrasound evaluation. *J.C.U.* 12 : 125, 1984.

Spertell, R. B., et al. Dysarthria-clumsy hand syndrome produced by capsular infarct. *Ann. Neurol.* 6 : 263, 1980.

Tepperman, P., et al. Motor speech disorders. *Postgrad. Med.* 68 : 86, 1980.

Victor, M., Hays, R., and Adams, R. Oculopharyngeal musculature dystrophy: A familial disease of late life characterized by dysphagia and progressive ptosis of the eyelids. *New Eng J. Med.* 267 : 1267, 1962.

Wertz, R. T. Neuropathologies of Speech and Language: An Introduction to Patient Management. In D. F. Johns (ed.), *Clinical Management of Neurogenic Communicative Disorders* (2nd ed.). Boston: Little, Brown, 1985.

Wolski, W. Hypernasality as the presenting symptom of myasthenia gravis. *J. Speech Hear. Disord.* 32 : 36, 1967.

Yorkston, K. et al. Perceived articulatory adequacy and velopharyngeal function in dysarthric speakers. *Arch Phys Med Rehab.* 70 : 313, 1989.

Yorkston, K., et al. Ataxic dysarthria: Treatment sequences based on intelligibility and prosodic considerations. *J. Speech Hear. Disord.* 46 : 398, 1981.

Yorkston, K. M., and Beukelman, D. R. A clinician judged technique for quantifying dysarthric speech based on single word intelligibility. *J. Commun. Disord.* 13 : 15, 1980.

Yorkston, K. M., and Beukelman, D. R. A comparison of techniques for measures of intelligibility of dysarthric speech. *J. Commun. Disord.* 11 : 499, 1978.

Index to Cases